PRAISE FOR *NUTRITION IN CRISIS*

"Fascinating book, full of original, interesting material by one of the original low-carb researchers whose grounding in the field goes back decades. Feinman combines a unique perspective with the experienced eye of a scientist. He's had a front row seat to developments in the field of carbohydrates and metabolism over the past decades, which has given him key insights into the latest research."
　　　　　—**Nina Teicholz**, author of *The Big Fat Surprise*

"With his usual cutting wit and verve, Dr. Feinman hacks through the tangled thicket of nutritional science to show us how we got to the sorry state we find ourselves in today, deploying his vast experience in biochemistry, nutrition, and the turgid mindset of academia to demystify mainstream nutritional research and explain how it has currently gone off the rails. With a sprinkling of humor and literary allusions, along with a deep dive into some of the nutritional literature, he tells readers what they need to know to shed excess body fat, lower blood sugar, and restore their health. A must-read for anyone with a serious interest in health and nutrition."
　　　　　—**Michael R. Eades**, MD, author of *Protein Power*

"We have arrived at the most important nutritional crossroads in all of human history: We must choose to either keep the dietary status quo despite every bit of evidence that it has failed, or demand a change in order to salvage what is left of our collective health. In *Nutrition in Crisis*, Dr. Richard Feinman has dropped the opening salvo in what is sure to be a battle for the ages—one that determines the future of how we eat and the prevalence of disease in the years to come. Join the revolution!"
　　　　　—**Jimmy Moore**, health podcaster; bestselling author of *Keto Clarity*

"Every scientific discipline needs a Dr. Richard David Feinman. He is just as skeptical about what he believes as what he disbelieves. His writing bears eloquent testimony to why he is such a scientific treasure."
　　　　　—**Timothy Noakes**, MD, PhD, emeritus professor,
University of Cape Town; founder, The Noakes Foundation

"As a physician who has worked with thousands of patients unraveling the mysteries and mythology around diet and nutrition, it is refreshing and timely to come across a sane voice among the misinformation perpetuated by a misaligned food industry.

We have moved far beyond the simple 'calorie in, calorie out' mentality and can now embrace biochemical individuality and updated research while avoiding the dogma of certain dietary camps."

—**Nasha Winters**, ND, FABNO,
author of *The Metabolic Approach to Cancer*

"I have devoted my medical career to normalizing blood sugars in people with diabetes. This is only possible with very low carbohydrate diets. Dr. Feinman explains why low-carb is wise even for people without diabetes. This can't-put-it-down title is the closest thing to a complete, popular analysis of the biochemistry of human nutrition that you will find and a superb lesson in how scientific studies have been manipulated to prove fiction."

—**Richard K. Bernstein**, MD, FACN, FACE, CWS,
author of *Dr. Bernstein's Diabetes Solution* and *The Diabetes Diet*

"Professor Feinman has been a leading pioneer in educating the academic community and lay public on the health benefits of low-carb and ketogenic diets for years. In addition to being a fantastic comprehensive review of practical nutritional biochemistry, his book also tells an informative and entertaining story about what went wrong in the nutrition establishment and advocates for a rational solution to the problem."

—**Dominic D'Agostino**, PhD, leading scientist
on ketogenic metabolic therapies

"Low-carb? Low-fat? Count your calories? If you have whiplash from trying to follow contradictory health headlines, you're not alone. We've gotten ourselves into quite a nutritional mess thanks to poorly done research that was even more poorly reported to the public. With his trademark wry humor, Dr. Feinman exposes just how shoddy much of the research has been and outlines how to take control of your own health."

—**Amy Berger**, MS, CNS, NTP,
author of *The Alzheimer's Antidote*

"A distinctively insightful treatise on the sad state of affairs in nutrition written by one of the true thought leaders. In his unique Brooklyn style, teacher and intellectual Dr. Richard Feinman fights against ignorance by enlightening people on the real science and application of nutrition."

—**Jeff S. Volek**, professor,
Department of Human Sciences, Ohio State University

"I've had the honor and privilege of knowing and working with Dr. Feinman for many years. I've watched him employ his deep knowledge of biochemistry and metabolism to tackle the entrenched, misguided nutritional advice cemented by thirty-five years of the food pyramid. His book says it all."

—**Eugene Fine**, professor, Department of Radiology,
Albert Einstein College of Medicine

"Dr. Feinman has spent his professional life dedicated to exposing the many flaws found in most reporting in nutrition science. *Nutrition in Crisis* walks the reader through the fog of dubious statistical analysis and into the light of day. In doing so Dr. Feinman examines the science behind the low-carb debate, using humor and metaphor to engage the reader in the process."

—**Miriam Kalamian**, EdM, MS, CNS,
author of *Keto for Cancer*

"Making the lifestyle and nutritional changes necessary for lasting health is difficult. *Nutrition in Crisis* supplies the intellectual imperative to take control of your own health without resorting to symptom-suppressing medication. Read it, learn *what* you need to do, and you will be mentally empowered and physically fortified for life!"

—**Dr. Sarah Myhill**, author of *Sustainable Medicine* and
Diagnosis and Treatment of Chronic Fatigue Syndrome and Myalgic Encephalitis

NUTRITION in CRISIS

Flawed Studies,
Misleading Advice,
and the Real Science of
Human Metabolism

Richard David Feinman, PhD

CHELSEA GREEN PUBLISHING

White River Junction, Vermont
London, UK

Originally published by NMS Press and Duck in a Boat LLC in 2014 as *The World Turned Upside Down: The Second Low-Carbohydrate Revolution*.

This edition published by Chelsea Green Publishing, 2019.

Acquisitions Editor: Makenna Goodman
Developmental Editor: Nick Kaye
Copy Editor: Deborah Heimann
Proofreader: Beth Kanell
Indexer: Linda Hallinger
Designer: Melissa Jacobson

Printed in Canada.
First printing February, 2019.
10 9 8 7 6 5 4 3 2 1   19 20 21 22 23

Our Commitment to Green Publishing

Chelsea Green sees publishing as a tool for cultural change and ecological stewardship. We strive to align our book manufacturing practices with our editorial mission and to reduce the impact of our business enterprise in the environment. We print our books and catalogs on chlorine-free recycled paper, using vegetable-based inks whenever possible. This book may cost slightly more because it was printed on paper that contains recycled fiber, and we hope you'll agree that it's worth it. Chelsea Green is a member of the Green Press Initiative (www.greenpressinitiative.org), a nonprofit coalition of publishers, manufacturers, and authors working to protect the world's endangered forests and conserve natural resources. *Nutrition in Crisis* was printed on paper supplied by Marquis that contains 100% postconsumer recycled fiber.

Library of Congress Cataloging-in-Publication Data
Names: Feinman, Richard D., 1940- author.
Title: Nutrition in crisis : flawed studies, misleading advice, and the real science of human metabolism / Richard David Feinman, PhD.
Description: White River Junction, Vermont : Chelsea Green Publishing, 2019.
Identifiers: LCCN 2018048431| ISBN 9781603588195 (paperback) | ISBN 9781603588201 (ebook)
Subjects: LCSH: Nutrition--Popular works. | Diet—Popular works. | Health--Popular works. | Diet in disease—Popular works. | Metabolism—Popular works. | BISAC: HEALTH & FITNESS / Nutrition. | MEDICAL / Endocrinology & Metabolism. | HEALTH & FITNESS / Diets. | HEALTH & FITNESS / Weight Loss. | HEALTH & FITNESS / Diseases / Diabetes. | HEALTH & FITNESS / Diseases / Cancer. | MEDICAL / History.
Classification: LCC RA784 .F45 2019 | DDC 613.2—dc23
LC record available at https://lccn.loc.gov/2018048431

Chelsea Green Publishing
85 North Main Street, Suite 120
White River Junction, VT 05001
(802) 295-6300
www.chelseagreen.com

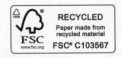

RECYCLED
Paper made from
recycled material
FSC® C103567

The book is dedicated to the memory of my father,
Max L. Feinman, MD,
who taught me about science and about honesty
and how much they were the same thing.

CONTENTS

Introduction

I've always had a weight problem. I would rarely have been considered fat, but I was always trying to lose weight. When I was eight years old, I wanted to get thinner so I could look sharp in my Brooklyn Dodgers uniform to impress Barbara Levy, who was the most beautiful girl in the world as far as I was concerned. I don't recall having any great success, and it was only fairly recently that I found out that Barbara Levy is now Barbara Boxer, former senator from California. In any case, I always knew that starch made me fat—oddly, I was less afraid of sugar because I mistakenly believed that there wasn't that much in Coca-Cola and the other sodas I drank. I grew up with what is usually called a poor self-image, and as the old joke goes, inside of every Botero is a Giacometti trying to get out.

I knew from early on that it was important to cut out starch and obvious solid sugar, and I made other observations about diet—for example, that cold cereal for breakfast made me slightly sick. It's difficult for me to remember exactly what I did eat in the morning. At least some of the time it was bacon and eggs, which, in those days, was just one of the things that people ate. Nobody recoiled in horror at bacon. The only dietary advice at the time was to eat from the different food groups, which were represented by a pie chart with unique symbols in each slice. The bottle of milk was one that stuck in my mind. I felt early on that it was not interesting, and I was sure that I didn't need an "expert" to tell me what to eat. When the USDA food pyramid was introduced, I knew it was a crock and I assumed that others did, too. My principles were simple: If you have a weight problem, bread will make you fat, and if you don't have a weight problem, why do you need the USDA? I thought everybody was in agreement on that, but obviously that wasn't the case. I'm not sure why people went along with all the "expert" advice. After all, everybody has a great deal of experience with food. We all do three experiments in "nutritional science" each day.

People's compliance with dietary standards probably has to do with the history of medicine. Among the turning points in that history was the discovery of vitamins. Unlike poisons and microorganisms, vitamins were stuff that you had to take if you didn't want to get sick. Another inflection point was the identification of cigarette smoke as a causal agent in lung disease. In that case, even though there was a toxic agent, the associations were subtle and one needed statistics or other expert insights to see the connection. This subtlety might have given people the idea that there were experts who could see harm where they couldn't.

In my youth, I simply ignored the "expert" advice. I thought that I knew what to eat (I was mostly right), and I saw obesity as a personal rather than professional question. Decades later, when I began teaching metabolism, I had to confront the interaction between science and nutrition. It proved to be more difficult than I would have guessed.

This book is the story of my encounter with the world of nutrition, a story of the science of biochemistry and metabolism—how you process the food that you eat. It is about the application of science to daily life, which is what I like about the subject. If you know a little chemistry, you can appreciate the way that human evolution has reached into the mixing pot of chemical reactions to obtain energy from the environment, and even if you don't know chemistry, you can see the beauty in the life machine.

But there is another side to the story. In the contentious and continually changing stories of nutrition in the media, I encountered a discouraging example of the limitations of human behavior in facing truth and preventing harm. The story of nutrition has proved to be an almost unbelievable tale of poor and irresponsible science within the medical community, one of the most respected parts of our society.

However hard it is for scientists to distrust experts, it is even harder for the general population. I was astounded when I saw a question on an online diabetes site that said, "My morning oatmeal spikes my blood glucose. How much carbohydrate should I have?" People with diabetes cannot adequately metabolize dietary carbohydrate (starch and sugar) so it seemed like an easy question. The answer from the experts, however, was waffling and tedious, and it didn't include the obvious advice: "Limit your oatmeal consumption to a level that doesn't spike your blood glucose."

Chemistry

When I was eight years old, my father taught me about atoms. I have one of those memories that might or might not be accurate: I am sitting in my father's car, and he is telling me that the whole world is made of atoms in the same way that the apartment building across the street is made of bricks. Whether or not the scene really took place, it was a major influence, and chemistry has long been a defining feature of my life. (Other vivid memories of my early life in Brooklyn—being at Ebbetts Field and seeing Jackie Robinson hit an inside-the-ballpark home run—turned out not to be true. He had hit only one, in 1948, before I had ever seen a live game).

The crux of atomic theory, the thing that captures everybody's imagination when they are first exposed to it, is that it is a global and absolute theory—it explains everything that has been done in the laboratory, the kitchen, or anywhere else. Various fields of chemistry get at that same sense of universal understanding with differing degrees of intellectual rigor, but eventually I recognized that biochemistry was a good place to be for a young person who didn't know what career he wanted to end up with. You can do drug design or theoretical chemistry or animal behavior or nutrition and still call yourself a biochemist.

Teaching Nutrition

I have worked in a number of fields in biochemistry, but it was teaching metabolism to medical students at SUNY Downstate Medical Center that led to my professional interest in nutrition. Metabolism is the study of the way food is processed and of the biochemical reactions that control life functions. It is a fairly complicated subject—those parts that we understand at all. Because there are so many individual biochemical reactions, students tend to see the subject in the same way that somebody once described the study of history: just one damn thing after another. There are general principles and big concepts, of course, but you do have to know the details. When I began teaching metabolism, I used the low-carbohydrate diet—at the time primarily a weight-loss diet—as a central element in my teaching. Control of blood glucose and insulin, the hormone whose release is controlled by glucose, is central to many different processes in biochemistry. In the complicated network of biochemical reactions, insulin stands out as a major point of regulation. The ups and downs of insulin are what we try to control through the use of dietary carbohydrate restriction as a therapeutic method. So, low-carbohydrate diets provided some unifying theme in teaching. I still teach metabolism in this way, though I now emphasize diabetes where impaired ability to handle dietary carbohydrate is the salient feature. The low-carbohydrate diet and its more thorough form, the ketogenic diet, are popular—periodically very popular—and while they remain controversial, the number of adherents, and possibly the desperation of the detractors, suggests that low-carbohydrate must inevitably be accepted as I will describe it: the "default" diet for diabetes (the one to try first) and the best diet for weight loss for many people. It is likely that its current popularity can't be turned back. Myself and others who use this teaching method have published papers about how understanding the real-world benefits of low-carbohydrate—getting control of your health and regulating your weight—can help you learn chemistry.[1]

Around 2000, one of our second-career medical students who had been a dietitian suggested that we include formal nutrition in our biochemistry course, and she provided subject matter from standard nutritional practice. I cannot really describe what it was about—probably, even at the time, it was so vacuous that I couldn't retain it in my memory. In any case, I objected because whatever it was, it wasn't biochemistry. The way I saw it, criticizing how lectures are given is like complaining about how the dishes are done: Everybody sees an immediate solution. Despite my protests, I wound up having to give formal lectures in nutrition, and I really didn't know the literature. I had long ago found that carbohydrate restriction was best for me, and while low-carbohydrate diets provided me with a good framework for teaching metabolism, applied therapies do not always have a close relation to theories, so teaching nutrition required a certain amount of background study on my part.

My first lectures on nutrition were neutral. I simply tried to cover the basic aspects of low-carbohydrate and low-fat diets—the two main choices, really—presenting the pros and cons of each approach in a simple way. Low-fat diets are not based substantially on biochemical mechanisms; instead, they follow from observed correlations between cardiovascular disease and the presence of cholesterol or other lipids in the blood.

More recently, low-fat has morphed into a prescription for obesity, and proponents have started emphasizing the point that fat has more calories per gram than other things, peddling the idea that the more calories, the greater the effect on body weight—the ill-conceived idea that "you are what you eat," which hangs over everything. While I could explain at that time how metabolism, and specifically the role of the hormone insulin, accounted for the benefits of a low-carb diet, I could not provide a well-organized review of the relevant studies in the medical literature. So, my initial lectures were rather simple and straightforward while I tried to get a grip on the scientific literature.

As I dug into that literature, however, it didn't take long to see that something was terribly wrong. In simply trying to grasp the facts, I had stepped into a world of bad science, self-deception, and a scandal equal to any in the history of medicine.

The Nurses' Health Study

Science is very specialized. Although I had been doing research on blood coagulation, which is related to cardiovascular disease (CVD), I did not pay much attention to the diet–heart hypothesis—the idea that fat and cholesterol in the diet raise blood cholesterol, which, in turn, leads to CVD. I was suspicious of such a theory, though, because biology tends to run on hormones and enzymes—that is to say, on control mechanisms rather than on mass action (the principle that chemical processes are determined by how much reactants are put into them). The grand principle in biochemistry is that there is hardly anything that is not connected with feedback. If you try to lower your dietary cholesterol, for example, your liver will respond by making more. Simply adding more or less is not guaranteed to produce much change at all, once feedback is taken into account. I was therefore skeptical, if not well-informed.

Whatever my misgivings about the diet–heart hypothesis, I didn't question it very deeply at first. However, when I went back to the original literature to find the evidence supporting low-fat recommendations, as I had to do in preparation for my lectures, it was a rude awakening. My assumption that there was at least a grain of truth in the diet–heart hypothesis turned out to be overly optimistic. If the hypothesis is not a

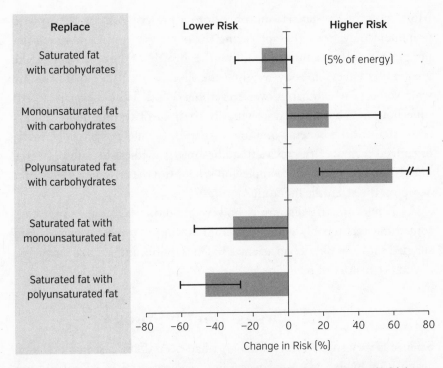

Figure 0.1. Estimated changes in risk of coronary heart disease associated with isocaloric substitutions (error bars show 95 percent confidence interval). Adapted from F. B. Hu et al., "Dietary Fat Intake and the Risk of Coronary Heart Disease in Women," *New England Journal of Medicine* 337, no. 21 (1997): 1491-1499.

total sham, it is pretty close. One of the first papers that I came across in my literature survey was a report from the Nurses' Health Study (NHS). Centered at Harvard, the NHS is one of the largest epidemiological studies with more than one hundred thousand participants. It has produced a large number of studies on nutrition and other aspects of lifestyle.

Walter Willett, head of the NHS and follow-up studies, and his associate Frank Hu examined the association of different kinds of fat, as well as carbohydrate, with the risk of CVD.[2] I found the result astounding. Figure 0.1, redrawn from their paper, shows the effects of substituting one type of fat for another, and of substituting carbohydrate for fat. Replacing saturated fat with either polyunsaturated fat (vegetable oils) or monounsaturated fat (olive or canola oil) reduced risk substantially. That's what the nutritional community had been saying, so I saw no surprise there.

However, when the polyunsaturated fat was replaced with carbohydrate, Hu et al. found an average 60 percent increase in risk. What? Carbohydrate is worse than fat for cardiovascular risk? That's not how it was supposed to be. What about saturated fat? Surely that's a bad guy. Replacing saturated fat with carbohydrate did provide some benefit according to the figure, at least on average, but there is more to the story. In this kind of figure, the error bars (horizontal lines) show the spread of individual values, which was quite large in this case. In other words, even though there was an *average* improvement from replacing saturated fat with monounsaturated fat—their main selling point—some subjects experienced greater benefit than the average, and some much less benefit than the average. When saturated fat was replaced by carbohydrate, some of the study's subjects were, in fact, going in the opposite direction—that is, they were at greater risk for CVD, which contradicted the supposed benefit of reducing fat. It wasn't just a few subjects, either. The breakdown was about 60:40: 60 percent of subjects experienced reduced risk of CVD by replacing saturated fat with carbohydrate, and 40 percent experienced greater risk. It gets worse. Without getting too caught up in the statistical details, the rule is that if the (horizontal) error bar crosses the zero line, then there is no significant effect of the substitution. So, based on the study's findings, substituting carbohydrate in place of saturated fat is at best neutral, or more precisely, it is as likely to increase risk as it is to lower it. The same is true of substituting carbohydrate for monounsaturated fat.

Looking at figure 0.1, it is hard to see a risk of fat, but hasn't risk from fat been the message all along? Certainly the idea that carbohydrate is a risk is not found in the media or the pronouncements of health agencies. And then there is the authors' summary of the paper:

> Our data provide evidence in support of the hypothesis that a higher dietary intake of saturated fat . . . is associated with an increased risk of coronary disease, whereas a higher intake of monounsaturated and polyunsaturated fats is associated with reduced risk. These findings reinforce evidence from metabolic studies that replacing saturated fat . . . with un-hydrogenated monounsaturated and polyunsaturated fats favorably alters the lipid profile, but that reducing overall fat intake has little effect.

This conclusion is not accurate. It's at best misleading, and at worst outright deceptive. The measured risk of saturated fat intake was dependent on what it was replaced with, yet there is no mention of carbohydrate as a replacement. The most striking thing to me was that if you looked at the risk from carbohydrate in comparison to the risk from saturated fat—that is, the risk of substituting one for the other—there was no difference. Even worse, substituting carbohydrate for other fats increased risk. How could this be? Fat out. Carbohydrate in. Wasn't that the clear recommendation for improved health from just about every health agency and expert? Yet the data said it didn't matter. Was it dishonest not to make this clear in the discussion section of the paper? At best, it was an error of omission. The authors from the Harvard School of Public Health were, and still are, the more modest among those vilifying fat, insisting that it is only the type of fat that we need worry about. Most recently, the American Heart Association (AHA) has come around to the same point of view as if they had just discovered it. I was probably not alone, but I began using the term *lipophobes* long ago for proponents of low-fat. It's a wiseguy term, and since I was still something of an inside player in the nutrition world, I was reluctant to put it into print until Michael Pollan started using it without any sense of irony.[3] (I started saying "…as Michael Pollan calls them.")

By the time I read the NHS paper, my professional involvement in the field of nutrition was cemented. I did not, however, adequately attend to the sense of being sucked into a whirlpool from which it would be hard to escape. The data supporting low-carbohydrate were there for everyone to see, I thought, even if the authors had chosen to downplay the strongest result.

A trip to the supermarket today demonstrates that the results from the Nurses' Health Study had little effect. The low-fat story is still with us. More striking is that two meta-analyses (averages of many studies) came to the same conclusion regarding the ineffectiveness of replacing fat with carbohydrate. Siri-Tarino et al. concluded that "there are few epidemiologic or clinical trial data to support a benefit of replacing saturated fat with carbohydrate," and in March of 2014, yet another meta-analysis found similar results.[4] What turned out to be most remarkable about all of these studies was that they presented a reanalysis of studies that had found no effect of saturated fat to begin with. One has to ask why the results were not accepted when first published. Some of the included studies are twenty years old. How is it possible that, in the most scientific period in history, our society runs on incorrect scientific information? That's one of the questions that I will try to answer in this book—or at least describe, as I'm not sure that there is a clear-cut answer. Looking ahead, I will introduce the revolutionary idea that, except in cases of well-defined genetic abnormalities, there is no predictable effect of diet on heart disease based on the current research. It is a hypothesis, and we might know more as we understand the genetics, but no effect is certainly more plausible than the diet–heart hypothesis, which remains only a conjecture without experimental support. This lack of effect will be one of the themes in this book and one of the battlegrounds as the crisis in nutrition plays out.

About This Book: Who It's for and Why I Wrote It

Food and chemistry have been two of the largest influences in my life. The beauty of biochemistry is that it relates the movement of electrons to what's on our plates—and this is a connection I thought I could explain. I like writing about biochemistry. It allows us to see how things fit together, but it also exposes the things we don't know—the things that evoke within us curiosity, the defining feature of the scientific life. If you want to indulge that curiosity, you are the person I had in mind when I started the book.

This is a book for scientists. Not specifically for people with atomic-force microscopes in their labs, but for those who want to look at nutrition from a scientific point of view. Science is less about sophisticated measurements than it is about basic honesty. It is true that scientific fields can be very mathematical or intellectually rigorous, but all sciences, even those as complex as quantum mechanics, are tied to logic and common sense, and are frequently directly accessible to lay audiences. Part of the game, most researchers understand, is to make the results easy to understand. Einstein is widely quoted as having said that we want to make it simple but not too simple. Modern medicine, despite its reliance on technology, explicitly accepts an obligation to explain things logically to the patient. It doesn't always fulfill this obligation well, but the goal remains nonetheless. In this book I will try to fill some of the gaps and define words, but for the tough spots, you will have to read like a scientist. How do we read? We're all specialists so most of us can't read technical articles, even those in our own fields, without some bumps. Skip over the bumps and see if you can get the big picture. You can always come back to them later, and many of the details are just a Google away.

If you write a book about biochemistry, it's about chemistry, but if you write a book about nutrition, it's about everything. Not every chapter in this book is for everybody. I have tried to provide a continuous, easy-to-follow thread, but different subjects require different kinds of discussion, and some of these discussions are necessarily technical. You can skip them, but I do suggest giving them a shot.

Although this is primarily a book about the science of nutrition, you can't escape the sociology and politics of medicine. Establishment medical journals, private organizations, and government health agencies have insisted on low-fat, low-calorie dogma despite the scientific evidence to the contrary. This politically motivated breakdown in scientific practice is deeply discouraging to me and was an additional motivation for my writing this book. The corruption of science goes beyond principle, too—what's at stake is the health of patients.

The breakthrough in understanding metabolism that underlies much of this book comes from the realization that many superficially unrelated pathologic or disease states and associated conditions are intimately connected at the physiological and biological level. Equally important, control of these states rests in a major way with diet. Diabetes, obesity, cardiovascular disease, states of hypertension, and numerous other physiologic states are all tied together. The promise is that, examined together, they might provide a global theory of metabolism and with it a common cure.

A major focus of this book is the concept of metabolic syndrome, which is a collection of clinical markers—including overweight, high blood pressure, and the so-called atherogenic dyslipidemia (the lipid markers that are assumed to contribute to cardiovascular disease)—that together and in combination indicate risk of disease. The identification of metabolic syndrome constitutes, in my view, a great intellectual insight. That the common effector is likely the hormone insulin points to the importance of controlling dietary carbohydrate, the major stimulus for insulin secretion.

The resistance of the medical profession to dietary carbohydrate restriction in the treatment of metabolic syndrome, and even more obviously, in the treatment of diabetes, I find incomprehensible. Everybody knows somebody with diabetes. Echoes of the early days in Brooklyn made it very upsetting to see pictures of Jackie Robinson taken shortly before his death from diabetes complications at age fifty-two. Because it is progressive, the disease is an underappreciated source of suffering. Clinicians will tell you that it is like cancer in its devastating effects. Diabetes is the major cause of amputations after accidents and the major cause of acquired blindness. That is a motivation for writing this book and why you might find it important.

This resistance is a scandal at the level of Ignaz Semmelweis, an early-nineteenth-century Viennese physician. To reduce the incidence of puerperal fever (infection after childbirth), Semmelweis suggested that physicians wash their hands after performing autopsies and before delivering babies. They refused; it was too much trouble. But that was the nineteenth century, before the germ theory was established, and that's some kind of excuse. It's hard to know how we will look back on the actions of the American Diabetes Association (ADA), who believe that for people with diabetes, "Sucrose-containing foods can be substituted for other carbohydrates in the meal plan or, if added to the meal plan, covered with insulin or other glucose-lowering medications."[5]

The most difficult part of writing this book was trying to understand—if such a feat is even possible—how the whole field of medical nutrition could be wrong. Way wrong. Totally off the mark. As misguided as the alchemists' pursuit of the creation of gold. This disconnect from true science is not only bizarre; it is a source of real harm to patients. The phenomenon is particularly hard to explain because the widespread respect for the medical professionals is based on real accomplishment and expertise, and it is hard to see why they would go so wrong in nutrition. For me, having precedents makes it easier to grasp, if not completely comprehensible. Here's one example of self-deception and refusal to accept evidence that I keep in mind. The following is a passage from Abraham Rabinovitch's writing on the Israel Defense Forces and intelligence in the days before the Yom Kippur War (1973):

> The intelligence chiefs believed they knew a deeper truth . . . that rendered irrelevant all the cries of alarm going up around them. Zeira and his chief aides were to demonstrate the ability of even brilliant men to adhere to an idée fixe in the face of mountains

of contrary evidence. . . . They clung to their view even though the Egyptian deceptions were contradicted by evidence of war preparations that AMAN's [military intelligence] own departments were daily gathering. . . . But the deception succeeded beyond even Egypt's expectations because it triggered within Israel's intelligence arm and senior command a monumental capacity for self-deception.[6]

The Israelis could have lost it all. They could have lost the whole country due to their refusal to accept the evidence. They were largely saved, however, by a couple of field commanders who were wild and crazy guys—most notably Ariel Sharon, who attacked an Egyptian emplacement by disobeying orders not to cross the Nile. Audacity and the refusal to follow orders might be what save nutrition as well.

Finally, this book is for the person (and those for whom she spoke) who posted on my blog wondering how she could determine which nutritional studies are flawed and which are not, especially at a time when we are inundated with so many conflicting recommendations. "Where are the true studies that are NOT flawed," she wrote, "and how do I differentiate?"

She was right to be suspicious. It is not always easy. There are so many nutrition papers that try to snow you with technical detail, and those are in fact the ones to be most suspicious of. Scientific papers will necessarily have technical components, but researchers shouldn't be making their results more difficult to understand than they need to be—and some of the papers are simply not true. Most researchers know that if you make up the data on a federally funded grant, you can go to jail, but when it comes to interpreting the data, they can say just about any damned thing. In this book, I explain how to interpret nutrition papers. In particular, I explain what the statistics mean, how they can be misused, and how to navigate the literature as someone who doesn't necessarily have a background in statistics.

The Second Low-Carbohydrate Revolution

The killer app, so to speak, of the low-carbohydrate diet is still the treatment of diabetes. Intuitively obvious, proved in many experimental trials, and widely used anecdotally and clinically, there are virtually no contraindications. Resistance to its use appears to be spurred on entirely by pressure from political organizations, primarily the American Diabetes Association (ADA), which, looking for a way to save face, still refuses to endorse low-carbohydrate strategies. Many identify the influence, direct or indirect, of drug companies and food companies as a culprit as well. Whatever the motivation, not encouraging physicians to at least offer carbohydrate restriction is seen by many who have had success with the approach as "criminal." The latest guidelines from the ADA emphasize "individualization," presumably as a way of softening their previous opposition to low-carbohydrate. The word *individualization* is used twenty-one times in their position paper,[7] but the actual principles to be applied for each individual are not stated. The foolishness of not explicitly restricting carbohydrate for people with a disease whose most salient manifestation is an inability to adequately metabolize carbohydrate is astounding. Individualization, in my view, can best be described as a cop-out.

Despite the resistance to low-carbohydrate, we have at the same time a constant flow of blog posts and books that show the low-fat diet–heart hypothesis for the intellectual and clinical disaster that it really is. The most recent and most complete, a book called *The Big Fat Surprise*,[8] is surprising in its description of the depths of self-delusion, if not dishonesty, in keeping low-fat alive. While the pace of criticism is increasing, these exposés document that the diet–heart hypothesis has been debunked since its inception.

If you step back and look at the data, the concerns, the voices on Huffington Post, or the numerous blogs belonging to dietitians, it shines through that the easiest way to lose weight is the low-carbohydrate diet. The concerns, voiced for forty years, have never been effectively substantiated, and the real-world tests of carbohydrate restriction come out in its favor. There are now dozens of successful implementations, though the Atkins diet is still the best known, having attained a somewhat generic status, like Kleenex.

Metabolic Syndrome: The Big Pitch

There is almost nothing in biology that is not connected with feedback. This idea is fundamental yet widely ignored. Reducing dietary intake of cholesterol will have limited effect because of compensatory synthesis.

Likewise, if you stop eating carbohydrate, your body will respond by synthesizing glucose and making other fuels available. This grand idea puts severe limitations on what you can do (as in the case of cholesterol or, looking ahead, trying to starve tumors by reducing glucose), but it also points to some opportunities. When you consume carbohydrate, the hormone insulin turns off the feedback system in the liver that produces glucose from glycogen or gluconeogenesis. Understanding that diabetes represents a breakdown in this feedback system—that the liver of a person with type 2 diabetes will not respond to insulin (insulin resistance)—makes clear why you should not add more insulin. Nonetheless, the compensatory feedback response to many drugs and foods does call for caution in jumping to conclusions.

The key point is that there is a global effect of the hormone insulin. We can get very far simply by regulating this hormone. The role of feedback is part of the picture, but the effects of manipulating insulin can be highly predictable, which is the main theme of this book. Always in the background of this discussion is metabolic syndrome (MetS). Metabolic syndrome is rooted in the observation, generally credited to Gerald Reaven, an endocrinologist who died recently, that a collection of seemingly different physiologic effects—overweight, high blood pressure, high blood glucose, high insulin, and the collection of blood lipid markers referred to as atherogenic dyslipidemia (high triglycerides, low HDL)—are all tied together by a common causal thread: disruption in the metabolic response to insulin.[9] The physiologic markers of MetS predict progression to the associated disease states (obesity, diabetes, hypertension, and cardiovascular disease), all of which respond to dietary carbohydrate restriction. That is the big pitch. This observation confirms that it really is a syndrome (since it has a common underlying cause) and simultaneously points us to the most effective treatment. No dietary approach is better than low-carbohydrate and no drug will target all of the markers together.

There are, in fact, critics of MetS who question the practical significance of the syndrome. What they're really suggesting is that the effects have to be treated with a collection of drugs: drugs for diabetes, drugs for heart disease, drugs for high blood pressure. A low-carbohydrate diet, which is already widely accepted as effective for weight loss, is likely *the* strategy to treat the different facets of MetS without using this cocktail of drugs. Acceptance of such a notion is the goal of the revolution.

Oddly enough, the bright light on the horizon is the ketogenic diet for cancer. I say "oddly" because carbohydrate restriction for diabetes is already a slam-dunk, and should have been the crystallizing point for change. Of course, as I've already discussed, the resistance to low-carbohydrate for people with diabetes has been extensive. Somehow treatment of cancer is not encountering the same obstinacy, despite limited research on the subject. In chapter 19 I describe work by my colleague Dr. Eugene J. Fine, targeting insulin in the treatment of cancer. I see this study, despite its small size, as a reason for hope and a sign of future progress.[10] If it turns out that we learn to treat diabetes by learning to treat cancer, it would not be the strangest thing that ever happened in science.

How to Approach This Book

If we had ham, we could have ham and eggs, if we had eggs.

—OLD AMERICAN IDIOM

This book represents the view of a practicing biochemist, and as such, it approaches nutrition as applied biochemistry. Biochemistry is not all there is to nutrition, but it represents a more scientific and logical perspective than "you are what you eat"; it tells us instead that we are what our metabolism *does* with what we eat. I will explain why low-carbohydrate diets are the default diet (the one to try first) for diabetes and metabolic syndrome and why you need to understand this idea even if you are not suffering from either condition. To be clear, I am not an advocate of anything. In the end, you have to be your own nutritionist. My job is to give you some tools for sorting out the army of nutritional "experts" out there and the studies they produce.

I am not an expert on politics, but, as in the aphorism most often attributed to John Adams (I think he stole it from the ancients), I study politics so that my children can study biochemistry and nutrition. It's all tied together. The science is not divorced from the politics. The Framingham Study,[11] the first very large population trial, tested not only a scientific principle—whether dietary fat and cholesterol were related to risk of cardiovascular disease (they were not)—but also whether the recommendations of health agencies were a rush to judgment (they were). The study had such a large political component that, as striking as the scientific outcome was—there was no effect of dietary total or saturated fat or cholesterol on cardiovascular disease—it couldn't be seen to fail. The results were buried for years until a statistician rediscovered them and finally had them published. This intertwining of the politics and science is a persistent pattern, and I try to tell both sides of the story and explain how they connect to each other.

My main principle, however, is that basic science comes first. I give preference to the demonstrations in nutritional and medical practice that are based in the fundamentals of biochemistry, of hard science. Big clinical trials have to be judged on their inherent strength, but, if they contradict basic science, the authors have an obligation to explain why. And science is continuous with common sense. It doesn't matter how many statistical tests you run: If the results violate common sense, it is unlikely to be science.

The poor research published by prestigious individuals and institutions suggests the nature of science itself has to be investigated. To do this, we will have to define scientific principles, explain how to read a scientific paper, and determine whether peer review has done its job. But first, in chapter 1, I give you the bottom line—the practical consequences of the science. The rest of the book will serve to justify these statements and recommendations.

PART 1

Setting the Stage

CHAPTER 1

Handling the Crisis

The Summary in Advance

What should I eat? This question invariably comes up during my lectures to medical students, during presentations at conferences, and even in private conversations about scientific experiments. Depending on my audience, I will go into different levels of technical detail, but the bottom line is always the same: The best diet is the one that works. Any expert can tell you how his or her diet theoretically conforms to widely accepted science, and how it is "healthy," "moderate," and a "bargain"—but if it doesn't work in practice, if you don't lose weight, if your blood sugar doesn't go down, then it's no good at all.

There is little evidence that the diets recommended by government and private health agencies have provided much help for the current epidemic of obesity and diabetes, but they keep pushing them anyway. Defenders usually tell you that it is because people are not really following the guidelines. What they don't say is how they know the recommendations are good if nobody follows them. So here I'll give you three basic rules of nutrition that I propose as a guide, and I'll show you a few principles that will help you follow them. My recommendations are likely different from what your doctor has told you. The rest of the book will justify these principles.

The Three Rules

The following are three simple, fundamental principles for getting control of your diet:

Rule 1. If you're OK, you're OK.

Rule 2. If you want to lose weight, don't eat. If you have to eat,
   don't eat carbs.
Rule 3. If you have diabetes or metabolic syndrome, carbohydrate
   restriction is the "default" approach—that is, the one to try first.

RULE 1. If you don't have a weight problem, if you feel OK, if you
are healthy, and if you don't have a family history of disease, there is
no compelling reason to change your diet. Rule 1 is actually surprising
to many people. You might want to find out more about nutrition and
biochemistry, but the idea that there was once a Garden of Eden diet that
we all ate until somebody first brought high-fructose corn syrup into the
world, along with all our woe, seems unlikely.

Not everybody has this view. There is the idea, not always stated explicitly, that, analogous to Freud's *The Psychopathology of Everyday Life*, we are
all doing something wrong and that life is a continuous battle between
what our bodies really need and the pressures of civilization. It's not like
that. We evolved to be adaptable. Lots of dietary approaches work and,
when it comes down to it, none of us are going to get out of this alive.

And then there are the Dietary Guidelines for Americans from the
USDA. Congress specifically charges the department with providing
advice to people who are healthy—that is, people who don't need advice. In
Brooklyn, we call this fixing something that ain't broke. Like psychoana-
lysts, these government nutritionists feel endowed by their Creator with
the intuitive power to penetrate unspoken, unmeasured, deep truths, and
believe that they are able to tell us that we are not eating the right thing and
that we are at risk for some future disease. They are, however, quick to take
offense if you suggest that their inability to control the epidemic of obesity
and diabetes makes it very unlikely that they know what the right thing is.

RULE 2. If you want to lose weight, don't eat. If you have to eat, don't
eat carbs. I first said this as a joke at a conference, but there is a great deal of
truth in it. This is not to say that starvation is a good long-term strategy—
the danger is that you will lose muscle mass along with your fat—but too
frequently we think that it is important to eat all the time. That is not true,
and intermittent fasting, which is garnering a certain amount of interest, might be a very useful strategy for weight loss. There are exceptions:
Some medical conditions, diabetes in particular, might require individual

variation. (Calorie reduction is beneficial for diabetes, but the need to avoid ups and downs means that there are other considerations.) The problem, though, is that we tend to think that hunger is some kind of physiologic signal telling us that our body needs food. We think that this signal must be answered immediately. It's not like that. Chapter 8 explains how hunger only means that you are in a situation where you are used to eating. This situation, such as a business lunch or a tailgate party, might have little to do with your state of nourishment. The hunger pangs that you feel might be real enough, but you are not compelled to answer them—and they don't even last that long.

Calories are a measure of the total energy available from burning food. The less food you eat, the less energy you will have. Not all calories are the same, though. Many experiments that show success with calorie reduction, on closer analysis, reveal that the effect was due to the de facto reduction in carbohydrate. Some dietary strategies will waste more energy than others (as heat and other unproductive effects). These nuances make up the second part of Rule 2, but the fundamental truth remains that if you don't eat, you will get thin.

RULE 3. If you have diabetes or metabolic syndrome, carbohydrate restriction is the "default" approach—that is, the one to try first. Almost everyone is now within two degrees of separation of somebody who has diabetes. Diabetes is a disease of carbohydrate intolerance. In type 1, there is a substantially reduced or total inability of the pancreas to produce insulin in response to carbohydrate. Type 2 is characterized by insulin resistance—the inability of the body's cells to properly respond to the insulin that is produced—as well as progressive deterioration of the insulin-producing cells in the pancreas. The defining symptom and major cause of the pathology is high blood sugar. The idea for treatment is simple: If diabetes is a disease of carbohydrate intolerance, it is reasonable to assume that adding dietary carbohydrate would make things worse, and restricting dietary carbohydrate would make things better. It makes sense, and this expectation is generally borne out. There are people with diabetes who can tolerate greater or lesser amounts of carbohydrate but, for most people, this simple treatment works exactly as it's supposed to—and dietary carbohydrate restriction might even be best for those people who can tolerate higher carbohydrate. There are no experimental or clinical data that show a contradiction. The fact that people with diabetes are not typically offered a low-carbohydrate diet as the default treatment, let alone as an option at all, is in my view a major scandal in the history of medicine.

Keep in mind that if you are on diabetes medication, you have to discuss getting on a low-carbohydrate diet with your physician. Carbohydrate restriction will lower blood glucose in the same way as many medications, so a low-carbohydrate diet in conjunction with your current medication regime might pose a risk of hypoglycemia (low blood sugar). Generally your physician, if he or she has any experience with carbohydrate restriction, will reduce or eliminate your medication before putting you on a low-carbohydrate diet. Some people see this as the single best argument for carbohydrate restriction: In most diseases, reduction in medication is considered a sign of success.

Doing It: Eat to the Meter

"Eat to the meter" is the principle used by people with diabetes. The meter is the glucometer, which, as you can probably guess, measures blood glucose. If the food you just ate causes a spike in blood sugar, it is a sign to avoid that food. Simple as that. Oddly, diabetes educators might tell you that if a food spikes your blood glucose, it means you need more insulin to deal with that food—a truly misguided notion.

Those of us with a weight problem might sensibly eat to what I call the ponderometer: the bathroom scale. If the experts tell you to eat more whole grains, but the reading on the scale keeps going up, then stop!

Doing It:
The Best Exercise Is the One That You Do

The nutrition world can't agree on much, but there are few who would dispute that exercise is inherently beneficial. Exercise by itself is not particularly effective for weight loss unless you're a professional athlete or in basic training, but it does enhance the benefits of dieting. Some of the effects are vascular—that is, physiologic rather than biochemical—so it is hard to pin down the relation to nutrition, but finding any agreement in this contentious field is a good thing.

A Brief Primer on Carbohydrate Restriction

Calories count, but the advice by experts that *only* calories count is wrong. There are great advantages to diet strategies that go beyond calories. For most people the best strategy for weight loss is to reduce carbohydrate intake. Insistence on the idea that "a calorie is a calorie," as it is usually stated, is one of the crystallizing points of the nutritional crisis. The benefits of a low-carbohydrate, higher-fat diet are due partly to the more satiating effects of protein and fat, or, more precisely, the poor satiation from most carbohydrate. It's important to keep in mind that "a calorie is a calorie" is not true as a general principle; instead, it is the macronutrient composition of the diet that affects the amount of weight gained or lost. There are extensive data in the medical literature to support the unique effects of carbohydrate reduction, but the best evidence might be anecdotal. In the field of weight loss, anecdotal evidence is actually fairly reliable. Everybody knows somebody who lost a lot of weight on the Atkins diet. Some report that the pounds seem to "melt away." There is no guarantee that you will have the same experience, and everybody hits a plateau, but it is still your best bet. Those who give dire warnings about low-carb diets likely haven't actually recommended them to patients or tried them personally.

Low-carbohydrate and ketogenic diets follow basic biochemistry. The key factor is improved control of insulin, the anabolic (building up) hormone that controls the major events in metabolism—storing fat and carbohydrate as glycogen, encouraging protein synthesis—and insulin is most reliably controlled by carbohydrate. Diets based on reduced carbohydrate are consistently successful and that's why people keep using them in the face of "concerns" of the medical establishment. As in any diet, people might quit at a certain point—we have six hundred million years of evolution and a lifetime of behavioral conditioning telling us to eat anything that tastes good—but even those who fall off the wagon will usually return to a low-carbohydrate diet. Nutritionists will tell you that "yo-yo dieting" has some risk, but there is no evidence for that, and most of us are happy for any period where we are thin, however long it lasts.

Whatever your concerns about low-carbohydrate, for most people, low-fat diets are even worse than doing nothing. The hunger will simply be too much to deal with. Sure, if you can get yourself into the frame of mind where you like the "lean and hungry" feeling, then anything that reduces calories will be okay. However, most people aren't able to deal with that feeling and will not be able to lose any significant amount of weight on a low-fat diet.

The scientific literature backs up the anecdotal evidence in support of low-carbohydrate. Jeff Volek, one of the major researchers in carbohydrate restriction, put this spin on it: "Nutrition research is hard. Too many things change and it's easy to come up with nothing. When you study low-carb diets, people lose weight. Put people on a low-carb diet and you get real data." As I finish this book, the long-standing refusal of the nutritional establishment to face the data is finally falling away. It will be increasingly easy to follow a low-carbohydrate approach and to have the support of a physician in doing so. Experimentally, carbohydrate restriction has better compliance than anything else because it gives immediate results, possibly due to the greater satiety of protein and fat, or, more likely, due to the poor satiety of most carbohydrates. You can test for yourself, at least at the level of perception.

Later chapters will describe experimental studies that support these conclusions about low-carbohydrate strategies, but there is one truly remarkable phenomenon that tells you about the edge low-carbohydrate diets have in satiety. When diet comparisons are carried out experimentally, most often the protocol is to allow the low-carbohydrate group the freedom to eat ad lib as long as they follow the restrictions on carbohydrate. Low-fat diets, on the other hand, are restricted to a fixed number of calories. The reason that the Atkins diet and other low-carbohydrate approaches put no limit on consumption is that fat and protein intake is self-limiting when carbohydrate is low. Setting up the experiment this way, however, constitutes poor experimental design because you are now testing two things: the ability of a low-carbohydrate diet to limit caloric intake as well as the proposed difference in physiologic effects of the type of diet—the metabolic advantage. The low-carbohydrate diet almost always wins in such comparisons, but because of the poor experimental design, you can't see how much of the success can be attributed to the greater satiety of low-carbohydrate diets as opposed to the greater weight loss per calorie. The results do tell you one thing, though: As advertised, you don't have to count calories in a diet based on carbohydrate restriction.

Perhaps the greatest virtue of carbohydrate restriction rests with its fail-safe feature. If you are not rapidly losing weight, or if you seem to hit the wall, it is a way of eating that gives you freedom from the sense of fighting a war against fat. You will almost never gain weight and you will escape that over-bearing feeling that every meal is a battle. This *feeling* might actually be the greatest threat of obesity. As a threat to health, excess weight is probably exaggerated. Mortality correlates with weight only at the very extremes. The major threat is the sense of loss of control. I am not a health care provider, but I get emails from executives, officers in the military, and other people who hold dominion over their professional world and who have trouble controlling their own body mass. The struggle can be a tremendous burden and can take over entire lives. Cut out most of the carbohydrates in your life, and you stand a chance of getting rid of the burden.

The best exercise, like the best diet, is the one that you can get yourself to do regularly. For that reason, exercise is highly individualized. Proponents of each type of exercise think that the others are not good, but the important thing is to find one that fits your style, or, more important, one that you get in the habit of doing. I am personally a believer in slow burn (slow repetition with heavy weights). This type of exercise is probably best for people who think that they are entering old age, in that it is efficient: You can get perceptible benefit from one set of ninety seconds.[1]

An encouraging development in exercise physiology is the technique called periodization, which is really just a pretentious way of saying that it is good to mix up different types of exercise on different days. You now have official sanction for switching between different types of exercise because you are bored.

Doing It:
Prepare for Battle, Prepare for Victory

Even the easiest diet has problems, ups and downs, and temptations. You have to plan out how you are going to handle different situations. If you know that the celebratory business meeting will be serving pizza, go in with a plan (eat beforehand, decide if you are comfortable enough to eat the toppings without the crust, etc.) There are techniques for staying on your diet and dealing with hunger, but you also have to prepare for success—that is, what to do if you actually aren't hungry. Suppose you've started a low-carbohydrate diet, you sit down to the recommended broccoli and steak, and you are full after eating one quarter of what you usually eat. You should be prepared to stop. In restaurants, doggie-bags are a good strategy unless you're on a first date, but then you'll probably be on your best behavior anyway. What should you do if the birthday cake looks disgusting and you don't want to eat it? It is, after all, your boss's birthday. There are many techniques. Put the birthday cake on your plate and walk around the room stabbing at it with your fork, for example. After a while you can set it on the sideboard with the other half-eaten pieces of cake. If you are worried about wasting food, ask for a doggie bag—tell them, "this is so good, but I can't eat another bite"—and then compost it when you return home.

Doing It:
Minister to Yourself, Cross-Examine the Experts

Doctor: Therein the patient
Must minister to himself.
Macbeth: Throw physic [medicine] to the dogs; I'll none of it.
—WILLIAM SHAKESPEARE, *Macbeth*

Doctors don't study nutrition. Nutritionists don't study medicine. Neither studies much science. This is an exaggeration, of course—many great scientists were trained as MDs—but it is not without some truth. Having an MD does not qualify a doctor on anything except their medical specialty. Experts have the obligation to justify their opinions, and you have the right to expect that justification. In the end, though, you are your own expert. Strive to learn as much as you can, and go for results rather than experts.

Perhaps most troubling is the proposition that the whole field of professional nutrition is fundamentally flawed. It is genuinely hard to understand how the progression of warnings about the lethal health effects of red meat or white rice can continue. These conclusions are not only contrary to our own intuitions, but when you look at the underlying data, they are actually scientifically meaningless. It is difficult to accept that the dozens of publications coming out of the Harvard School of Public Health and published in *The New England Journal of Medicine* are of extremely poor scientific quality. Where's the peer review? Where's the expert training? The failure of experts and the lack of genuine peer review represent a major component of the crisis in nutrition and in medicine at large. In this book I will give you the tools to see how establishment medicine went off track, and I will show you how the three rules will help you minister to yourself.

Doing It: The Low-Carbohydrate Principles

My personal preference is for principles over formal diets. However, if you like diets with precise instructions, there are millions. For low-carbohydrate and ketogenic diets, *The New Atkins for a New You*,[2] *Protein Power*,[3] and *The Art and Science of Low-Carbohydrate Living*[4] are good places to start. Paleo diets might also be of interest—they are like the Mediterranean diet in that nobody really knows what they are, but they are generally low-carbohydrate and employ a higher ratio of science to emotion than other options. Numerous books and websites will give you precise instructions and recipes for any of these diets. If your MO is to just fit the general low-carbohydrate strategy to your own lifestyle, on the other hand, these are the big principles.

Your Carbs Come from Vegetables

The simplest way to break into carbohydrate restriction is by brute force: no rice, no potatoes, no bread, no pasta, and no dessert beyond a small amount of fruit. What you have to sacrifice is dependent on your current diet. If you normally eat a steak with potatoes and broccoli, leave out the potatoes. This might be all you have to do. If you are full from this smaller amount of food, put the rest in the refrigerator, or compost it if it's going bad. If you still have an appetite, you can have more steak, but in fact most people don't want more steak even if they can afford it—so it's usually more broccoli. Vegetables contain some carbohydrate, but the important thing is that you don't really have to count anything. You are likely to have real success with this simple approach. If you have diabetes or metabolic syndrome, you are virtually guaranteed to get better—although, again, if you are taking medication, you have to do this with a physician who can lower your medications appropriately.

To delve a bit deeper, you need to understand a couple of things: First, there is a graded response, which means that the benefit is roughly proportional to the amount of carbohydrate that you remove from your eating; and second, there is a breakpoint, where there is enhanced weight loss. The breakpoint is generally marked by the presence of ketone bodies in the blood (ketosis) and urine. Strictly speaking, the presence of ketone bodies in the urine is called ketonuria (although frequently taken as a sign of ketosis). The ketone bodies indicate a significant switch from reliance on carbohydrate as an energy source to a new, predominantly fat-based metabolism. At this point, you will have to attend more precisely to how much carbohydrate you actually ingest. The simple rules above will likely get you in the carbohydrate range of 100 grams per day, which is a big switch for most Americans. To go into ketosis, you will have to go below 20–50 grams per day, though different people have different cutoffs.

Though the Atkins diet has assumed the status of Kleenex and is considered the generic low-carbohydrate diet, it actually has a more specific strategy than you might realize. The Atkins diet's recommendation is to achieve ketosis for two weeks, followed by gradually re-adding carbohydrate into the diet, presumably for reasons of taste or possibly on the principle that you want to eat similarly to how you used to but without making yourself fat. Many people stay in ketosis indefinitely, but this requires more attention and usually a period of adaptation.

My survey of an online support group called the Low-Carber Forums[5] found that the majority of people on low-carbohydrate diets eat all the nonroot vegetables they want without counting grams of carbohydrate, even though most of these individuals thought that they were on the Atkins diet, which specifies precise grams of carbohydrate.

If you eat at home a lot, it is important to learn how to cook vegetables. Like many tasks, cooking vegetables involves spending a great deal of time thinking and procrastinating and a relatively small amount of time actually doing the job. A good solution is to time yourself—the task likely ends up taking less time than you'd imagined. So, find the appropriate vegetable dishes for either quick cooking or for cooking in advance. Cauliflower, for example, is a common component of low-carbohydrate diets, and you can make steamed cauliflower in just a few minutes. Eat it straight or use it later for other very quick recipes.

Don't Be Afraid of Fat

People have always eaten fat. The antifat campaign is of recent origin, and countless histories and exposés have proven its lack of grounding in scientific evidence. It has been one of the truly bizarre phenomena in the history of science—in this most scientific of periods, we have simply ignored the failures of the numerous experimental trials of the low-fat idea. The big clinical studies—the Framingham Study, the Oslo Diet Heart Study, and a dozen others culminating in the Women's Health Initiative—have found no support for the theory. When pressed, most health agencies say that there is nothing wrong with fat in general, only with saturated fat, but even the evidence for removing saturated fat is missing from the big studies.

From the scientific point of view, however, these studies were successful. They asked the real question: "Are low-fat, especially low-saturated-fat, dietary patterns beneficial for prevention of cardiovascular disease and other health problems?" Many were well done, within the limitations of large population studies, and they gave a clear answer: No. Low-fat diets, especially low-saturated-fat dietary patterns, do not provide benefit. A clear question was posed and the answer was equally clear. Of course, as in court, you cannot be found innocent, only not guilty. There might well be conditions where saturated fat is a risk, but we have not found them. We suspect that high saturated fat in combination with high carbohydrate might have risk but we haven't even been able to show that.

So, my advice—grounded in the existing evidence—is to not be afraid of fat. If you are concerned about saturated fat, there are numerous alternatives, but I would not advise trying to go low-carbohydrate *and* low-fat unless you like being hungry. You might, in fact, like the feeling—feelings are different if we impose them ourselves rather than having them imposed on us. Total calorie restriction does have general health benefits, but, even there, the de facto reduction in carbohydrate is likely the controlling factor.

Desserts and Sweets

Carbohydrates as a chemical class encompass simple sugars and their polymers, starch and related compounds. Reducing sugar intake is part of reducing carbohydrate intake, and sugar is an easier target for elimination than other sources of carbohydrate: Candy is considered frivolous. Because sugar assumes a more discretionary position, it might be the best place to start reducing carbohydrate intake, and for some people, elimination of sugar might be all that's necessary. It's important that you don't put starch back in place of the sugar that you remove, though. What the strange collection of bedfellows currently involved in the political movement that I call fructophobia, the attack on sugar, forgot to tell you is that sugar is a carbohydrate. If you cut out sugar and replace it with "healthy" high-grain, high-carbohydrate oatmeal, you are stacking the cards against yourself (even if you think that oatmeal offers benefits in fiber that offset the number of carbohydrates). Many people, anecdotally, gain benefit by simply removing sugar-sweetened soda, but if you have a sweet tooth, you might need some help. One strategy is to imagine that you are conducting an experiment. The hypothesis from anecdotal observation is that cravings for sweets disappear after three days without sweets. Your experiment will test whether that is true for you.

If you must have something sweet, there are several nonnutritive sweeteners—some natural, some artificial. You might want to avoid artificial sweeteners, however, especially those in diet soda, because they can sustain your taste for sweets and provoke bad reactions in certain individuals. The scare stories about the artificial sweeteners are not scientifically sound, but the possible psychological effect of "sweetness" might be real.

You should do whatever works for you, but I think that for most people, it is best to avoid the common nutritional advice that you are allowed treats or that you are allowed a cheat day. You are not allowed treats. Nobody's perfect and sweet things do taste good, and you will have some. We all screw up periodically, and when this happens, you just have to get back to the plan. However, sweets are not allowed in the sense of being a specific feature of your diet. Consumed sweets are, scientifically speaking, experimental error. There are people who are able to incorporate some sweets as part of their diet, who don't deviate from the single ice-cream bar that they have every day as their lone large source of carbs. Some people can get away with eating these sweets, and if you like food, you will certainly find foods that are worth the risk to your diet, but they are not allowed in the sense of a recommendation. There is a big difference between the attitude that you can't be perfect and the attitude that you deserve an occasional treat. But I am not suggesting that you should indulge feelings of guilt or mentally beat yourself up. The psychologist Alfred Adler always advised: "Do the wrong thing or feel guilty but not both."

The current hysteria about sugar might help you cut back, but there is great danger in characterizing things as forbidden fruit, as our very earliest history shows, especially when someone is trying to ban that forbidden fruit. Being told that you can't have something might make it more appealing, and when you see the absurd lengths that the media and researchers alike go to in order to demonize sugar, you might begin to think it is safe. Lawyers call this the Reverse Mussolini Fallacy: Just because Mussolini made the trains run on time doesn't mean you want them to be late. (The last time I was in Italy, the trains did run on time, contrary to the Italian stereotype.) Just because the USDA says it's bad, doesn't mean it's good.

Fruit and Other Tricky Foods

All fruits contain sugar, and as with any type of food, it is best to stay with the rule: Eat to the meter. If it doesn't interfere with weight loss or blood sugar, or whatever your goal is, then it is OK. I like Suzanne Somers's technique. Unlike many experts who might be thin themselves (what does Walter Willett know about fighting fat?), Somers lost a part in *Starsky and Hutch* because they told her she was "a little too chunky." She recommends eating fruit in pieces—half an apple now, the other half later—with the goal of avoiding insulin spikes.[6]

Mike and Mary Dan Eades, authors of *Protein Power*, ran a clinic for many years. They had thousands of patients on low-carbohydrate diets. Despite generally achieving great success, they had several patients who complained that they had faithfully adhered to the diet but were not losing weight. The Eades found that the three most common foods that caused trouble were cheese, nuts, and nut butters. When these were reduced or removed from the (already low-carbohydrate) diet, patients were able to continue to lose weight. Cheese is probably a simple matter of overconsumption. Although apparently safe, moderation must be applied to cheese. Dr. Atkins recommended that you restrict yourself to hard cheeses,[7] which pretty much means serious cheeses that you might find in a gourmet cheese shop. Although it's not obvious what was behind his recommendation, the greater intensity might be more satisfying, and the current price of good cheese (e.g., two- or three-year aged Gouda) also ensures moderation for most of us.

"Not a License to Gorge"

The phrase "not a license to gorge" appears in the original Atkins book several times.[8] The idea is that, although there are no stated limits on what you can eat as long as you keep carbohydrate low, overeating is not encouraged. The principle that "a calorie is a calorie" is not correct, but calories do count, and if you are concerned about your weight, you undoubtedly already know that it is possible to defeat any diet. The nutritionists usually give you exactly the wrong advice but are actually right about eating slowly. Satiety sets in slowly. For people who like food, the prescription is simply to not eat if you are not hungry. A possible exception is a situation where you feel that you have the kind of cravings that will set your low-carbohydrate diet back. In such a case it might be useful to eat something that's allowed to satiate the craving, even if it seems like overeating: some high-protein, high-fat food (if you have an Eastern European butcher, real kielbasa is best). Eventually, your cravings will stabilize. In general, the corollary to the second part of Rule 2 is that if you have to overeat, don't overeat carbs.

Diet Definitions

There are many variations of diets based on carbohydrate restriction. As a treatment for diabetes, the principle is to keep carbohydrate as low as possible. In less stringent conditions, there might be more room for

Table 1.1. Operational Definitions of Carbohydrate-Restricted Diets

Diet	Carbohydrate restriction
Very low-carbohydrate ketogenic diet (VLCKD)	20–50 grams per day, or less than 10% of the 2,000 kilocalories per day diet. Generally, although not always, accompanied by ketosis, this is the level of the early phases of the plans in many popular carbohydrate books.
Low-carbohydrate diet	Less than 130 grams per day, or less than 26% of a nominal 2,000 kilocalories per day diet. This corresponds to the ADA definition of 130 grams per day. This is a generally accepted number, likely derived from misinterpretation of Cahill's study of the onset of ketosis.
Moderate-carbohydrate diet	26–45% of the 2,000 kilocalories per day diet. The upper limit is chosen as the approximate carbohydrate intake before the obesity epidemic (43%). Current consumption is about 49%.
High-carbohydrate diet	Greater than 45% of the 2,000 kilocalories per day diet. Recommended target on ADA websites. The 2015 Dietary Guidelines for Americans recommend 45–65% carbohydrate.
For comparison	
Pre-obesity epidemic (1971–1974– NHANES I)	Men: 42% carbohydrate (~250 grams for 2,450 kilocalories per day) Women: 45% carbohydrate (~150 grams for 1,550 kilocalories per day)
Year 1999–2000	Men: 49% carbohydrate (~330 grams for 2,600 kilocalories per day) Women: 52% carbohydrate (~230 grams for 1,900 kilocalories per day)

maneuvering. If specific diets are referred to, table 1.1 provides the associated guidelines that have been published in several peer-reviewed journals by professionals with the credentials and experience.

These definitions are important. Authors in the nutritional literature give themselves license to call anything that they want a low-carbohydrate diet. With a straw man in hand, it is not hard to show that a low-carbohydrate diet is dangerous to your health, but the results have very little to do with the actual established guidelines.

Depending on your goal and who you are, you might experience a graded response: The greater the carbohydrate reduction, the greater the weight loss, and the greater the improvement in blood glucose. Particularly in weight loss, however, there might be a threshold effect. The onset of ketosis, which for most people occurs at a daily intake of about 30 grams, will have a more dramatic effect.

CHAPTER 2

Whaddaya Know?

For several years, we gave incoming medical students a questionnaire to assess their knowledge of nutrition. These students were among the most accomplished in the country, but, like everybody else, most of their nutritional information came from rumors and the fronts of packages on supermarket shelves. We didn't keep any quantitative feedback on the quiz, but some of students liked the format, and you might, too. No particular knowledge is assumed beyond your life experience as a nutritional end user, an eater. The quiz only tests how you were able to sift through all the information that's available on the internet and in popular books, and it is intended as a teaching device: The answers provide basic information. I provide the quiz first so you can see how you do, and then, as I go through the answers, I will delve into the nutritional concepts associated with each question. So, whaddaya know?

1. The most energy-dense food (most calories per gram) is:

   ☐ carbohydrate   ☐ protein
   ☐ fat   ☐ alcohol

2. For a slice of buttered bread, which is more fattening?

   ☐ the butter   ☐ You cannot tell from the
   ☐ the bread   information given.
   ☐ Both are equally fattening.

3. During the epidemic of obesity and diabetes, the macronutrient that increased most was:

   ☐ carbohydrate   ☐ All were about the
   ☐ protein   same. Calories increased
   ☐ fat   across the board.

4. The macronutrient most likely to raise blood glucose in people with type 2 diabetes is:

☐ carbohydrate   ☐ fat
☐ protein   ☐ alcohol

5. The dietary requirement for carbohydrate is:

☐ approximately   ☐ as much as possible
   130 grams per day   ☐ There is no dietary
☐ approximately   requirement for
   50 percent of calories   carbohydrate.

6. The amount of carbohydrate recommended by the American Diabetes Association and other health agencies is:

☐ approximately   ☐ as much
   130 grams per day   as possible
☐ approximately   ☐ as little
   50 percent of calories   as possible

7. A good source of monounsaturated fat is: (check all that apply)

☐ butter   ☐ avocado oil   ☐ flaxseed oil
☐ olive oil   ☐ corn oil
☐ canola oil   ☐ soybean oil

8. The diet component that is most likely to raise triglycerides (fat in the blood) is:

☐ fat   ☐ carbohydrate   ☐ protein

9. In general, what effect does a low-fat diet have on HDL-C (high-density lipoprotein cholesterol, i.e., "good cholesterol")?

☐ increase   ☐ decrease   ☐ no change

10. The dietary change that is most likely to increase the risk of cardiovascular disease is:

☐ unsaturated fat   ☐ unsaturated fat   ☐ carbohydrate →
   → saturated fat   → carbohydrate   unsaturated fat

☐ carbohydrate   ☐ saturated fat   ☐ saturated fat →
→ saturated fat   → carbohydrate   unsaturated fat

The Calorie, the Calorimeter

Now that you've taken the time to complete the quiz, let's see how you actually did. I encourage you to keep a tally as you go along and see how you stack up against the incoming medical students.

1. The most energy-dense food
   (most calories per gram) is: **Student response (%)**

   ☐ carbohydrate   11
   ☒ fat   85
   ☐ protein   4
   ☐ alcohol   0

Our first-year medical students do surprisingly poorly on the first question, considering how basic it is. Typically only 85 percent of our incoming class gets it right. Although they have not yet been through the metabolism course, this is a highly educated group of people, so you would assume that everyone knows that fat is the most energy-dense macronutrient. The likely explanation is that they are not curious about nutrition because they don't see it as part of medicine and because they are mostly young, healthy, and thin.

The operational numbers in kilocalories per gram are 4, 4, 9, and 7 for carbohydrate, protein, fat, and alcohol, respectively. Calories are a measure of energy, and calories in nutrition represent the energy that we can obtain by metabolizing ingested food. In physics, energy is defined as the ability to do work, which is not so different from the common day-to-day idea. By using a device called a calorimeter to measure heat—one form of energy— we are able to determine the total number of calories in a sample of food. The food is placed in a small container in an atmosphere of oxygen under pressure, and it is then ignited. The container is surrounded by a water bath that heats up when the sample is ignited. By recording the change in temperature in the water bath, we can calculate the amount of heat generated from the combustion, and this number can be assigned to the oxidation of the food. This is the real definition of the nutritional calorie.

In physics, the definition of a calorie is given as the amount of heat required to raise the temperature of water by one degree. The dietary "calorie" is equal to a physical kilocalorie (kcal)—that is, 1,000 physical calories. Use of "kcal" in nutrition is increasing, and in this book we use kcal when referring to quantity for the sake of clarity. This is one small step toward helping nutrition become scientific.

The definition I have given for a calorie is quite simple, but there are some very important nuances: The calories assigned to a food represent the energy for complete combustion of that food in oxygen. Calories refer to the following chemical reaction, not to the food itself:

$$Food \; + \; Oxygen \; \rightarrow \; Carbon \; Dioxide \; + \; Water$$

$$or$$

$$Food \; + \; O_2 \; \rightarrow \; CO_2 \; + \; H_2O$$

Heat produced in the calorimeter measures the energy for this specific reaction. Again, the energy is in the reaction, not in the food. It is not like particle physics where the mass of a particle is given in units of electron-volts, a measure of energy, (because of $E = mc^2$). We will come back to this point when we delve into thermodynamics and consider what is wrong with the idea that a "calorie is a calorie" in chapter 9.

Fat is the most energy-dense macronutrient at 9 kcal per gram (kcal/g), and for that reason, it is considered inherently fattening by nutritionists. This is the basis of traditional recommendations for low-fat diets for obesity. There is more to the problem than caloric density, however, and it turns out that there is more to getting fat than total calories. To see how this all plays out in a real situation, consider the next question.

2. For a slice of buttered bread,
    which is more fattening?   **Student response (%)**

☐ The butter.	11
☐ The bread.	85
☐ Both are equally fattening.	4
☒ You cannot tell from the information given.	0

While we do not normally ask trick questions, this falls into that category. An argument could be made that because butter has an energy density of 9 kcal/g, it is inherently more fattening, but you really need more information. If you put a lot of butter on the bread, it would indeed be more fattening, but in fact, people rarely put more than one tablespoon of butter (approximately 100 kcal) on a slice of bread (also approximately 100 kcal). Yes, fat is the most calorically dense food, but caloric density, like any density, can be very misleading: Density is a measurement per amount of material—per unit of volume, per gram, per something—so it matters how much of that something you actually have. Calories per gram is not informative unless you know how many grams. Things like caloric density, or any density for that matter, are measures of intensity, and technically are called intensive variables. An intensive variable does not depend on how much you have: One tablespoon of butter has the same energy density (kcal/g) as two tablespoons of butter, but obviously two tablespoons have twice the total calories. Such total, absolute measurements are called extensive variables. It's like that riddle: Which is heavier? A pound of uranium or a pound of Styrofoam? Of course they are the same. A pound is a pound. Uranium has an extremely high density (about 1.6 times that of lead), so a pound of uranium is only a little bigger than a major league baseball, whereas a pound of Styrofoam would fill up an entire room.

Fraction, or percent, is another kind of measure of intensity that can be misleading. Looking ahead, this is one reason that providing the percent increase of risk in a clinical test is not helpful, however much the media and scientific literature might seize on such numbers. After all, your odds of winning the lottery are increased by 100 percent, or doubled, by buying two tickets instead of one—but should that really make you want to play? Bottom line: When you hear people say that fat has more calories per gram, know that it is irrelevant. You have to know how many grams you are actually eating.

The Obesity Epidemic

So, what did we eat during the obesity epidemic of the past thirty or forty years? What kinds of macronutrients were in our diet? You might know this better than our students, who probably did not attend to the problem.

3. During the epidemic of obesity and diabetes,
   the macronutrient that increased most was: **Student response (%)**

   ⊠ carbohydrate   53
   ☐ protein   4
   ☐ fat   2
   ☐ All were about the same.   41
   Calories increased across the board.

At this point many students have caught on to where I'm coming from, and there are probably more votes for carbohydrate than if this had been the first question. However, many people, students included, still think that calories increased across the board. The epidemic of obesity and diabetes has been accompanied by a substantial decrease in the percentage of fat in peoples' diets, and, at least for men, the absolute amount of fat consumed also went down slightly.

Figure 2.1 shows data from the National Health and Nutrition Examination Survey (NHANES), which was conducted at the intervals listed on the horizontal axis. The vertical axis is the absolute amount of calories consumed, and the large increase in energy consumed appears to be due entirely to a dramatic increase in the consumption of carbohydrate. The percent change shown along the top indicates the expected decrease in fat, but, at least for men, the absolute amount of fat (total calories) and, notably, the absolute amount of saturated fat went down. (The extent to which this gender difference plays out in real life is not clear. Anecdotally, it is easier for men to lose weight, but the major effects of metabolism are qualitatively the same across sexes, and the benefit of controlling the glucose–insulin axis applies to women as well. Obviously, other hormones might play a role.)

There remains a lot of error in these kinds of surveys, but it is quite clear that there was no increase in fat intake. The clearest conclusion is that an increase in carbohydrate consumption, rather than fat consumption, is associated with greater total intake, and that a "Western diet," as they call it in the nutrition literature, does not mean a high-fat diet. It is widely said that association does not imply causality. The more accurate statement is that association does not *necessarily* imply causality. Few people would deny that the association of dietary calories and body mass is causal, however nonlinear the association might be. Whether the association

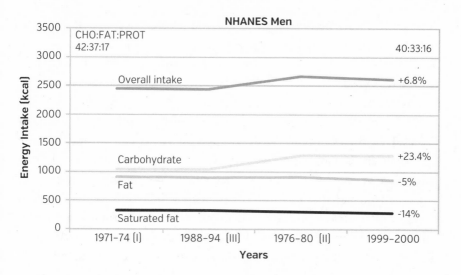

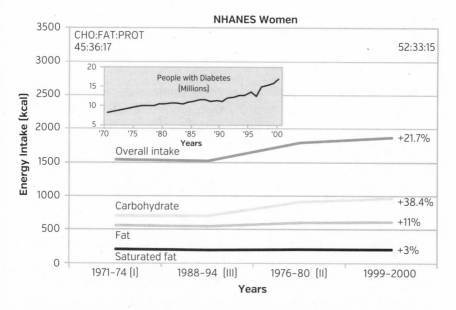

Figure 2.1. Consumption of macronutrients during the epidemic of obesity and diabetes. The horizontal axis represents the periods in which data was collected. The left vertical axis is the absolute energy input in kilocalories. The numbers on the far right refer to the percent change in calories. The ratios of macronutrients are shown along the top. *Note*: CHO = Carbohydrate. Data from the National Health and Nutritional Examination Survey.

between increased carbohydrate intake and increased calories is causative is one of the central questions explored in this book. The argument will be that, given the effectiveness of low-carbohydrate, high-fat diets as a treatment and sometimes a virtual cure for diabetes, it would be surprising if carbohydrate was not involved in some causative role.

Finally, there is an obvious association between the official advice of the USDA, the AHA, and other authorities to reduce fat and increase carbohydrates, and what people actually did. They reduced fat, at least as a percentage of calories, and they dramatically increased carbohydrate.

Looking ahead, one way to test whether there is a causal link between carbohydrate intake and obesity is to simply reduce carbohydrate under conditions of fixed calories while monitoring weight and incidence of diabetes. There are some good experiments that test this (see descriptions of Volek's experiment in chapters 7 and 11). Whatever else can be drawn from the NHANES data, the association between increased carbohydrate/decreased fat intake and obesity and diabetes is the single result that makes the largest impact on our medical students, and it remains an undercurrent in any analysis of the role of macronutrients.

4. The macronutrient most likely to raise blood glucose in people with type 2 diabetes is:	**Student response (%)**
☒ carbohydrate	83
☐ protein	Not available
☐ fat	Not available
☐ alcohol	Not available

This question is, or should be, obvious. The correct answer was chosen by 83 percent of our students. Statistics on the wrong answers were lost, but the surprise is that anybody got it wrong. Diabetes is fundamentally a disease—or, really, several diseases—of carbohydrate intolerance. Glucose normally stimulates secretion of the hormone insulin from beta cells of the pancreas. Insulin is a kind of master hormone, controlling fat and protein metabolism as well as maintaining normal blood glucose, and in that sense, carbohydrate controls other aspects of metabolism. People with type 1 diabetes cannot produce insulin in response to blood glucose. People with type 2 diabetes have progressive deterioration of the beta cells. They do produce insulin but their cells respond poorly—a phenomenon called insulin resistance. Diabetes is as much a disease of fat metabolism as of carbohydrate metabolism: The primary effect of insulin is on synthesis and breakdown of fat, and a person with type 2 diabetes might have excessive fatty acids in their blood. Nonetheless, the most obvious characteristic and the major cause of other symptoms remains the hyperglycemia (high blood glucose). Different carbohydrate-containing foods raise blood glucose to different extents, but the general principle holds that carbohydrate is the primary influence on blood glucose in people with diabetes.

The Dietary Requirement for Carbohydrate

There is no requirement for dietary carbohydrate as there is for the so-called essential amino acids or essential fatty acids. This does not mean that I recommend doing without them altogether, even if this were possible (it isn't: even meat has a small amount of carbohydrate).

5. The dietary requirement for carbohydrate is: **Student response (%)**

☐ approximately 130 grams per day	22
☐ approximately 50 percent of calories	32
☐ as much as possible	0
☒ There is no dietary	26
requirement for carbohydrate.	

The fact that there is no dietary requirement for carbohydrate means, in a practical sense, that if you do want to reduce carbohydrate, there is no biological limit on how much you can restrict the intake. The extent to which you actually do restrict carbohydrate intake will depend on your personal reaction and taste, but you do not *need* to consume any at all. Nutritionists will emphasize that the brain needs glucose, but your body is capable of making glucose from protein through the process known as gluconeogenesis and supplying glucose from storage as glycogen. There are also alternative fuels available in the form of ketone bodies. If you did need dietary carbohydrate, you would die if you went without food for a week—after all, you store a lot of fat but not much carbohydrate. I write more on glycogen and gluconeogenesis in chapter 5.

6. The amount of carbohydrate recommended
by the American Diabetes Association and
other health agencies is: Student response (%)

☐ approximately 130 grams per day   33
☒ approximately 50 percent of calories   35
☐ as much as possible   0
☐ as little as possible   30

It is hard to believe that a diabetes agency would recommend any significant amount of carbohydrate, yet their 2008 dietary guidelines contain the rather remarkable advice that "Sucrose-containing foods can be substituted for other carbohydrates in the meal plan or, if added to the meal plan, covered with insulin or other glucose-lowering medications. Care should be taken to avoid excess energy intake. (A)"[1]

The truth is that starch, which is a polymer of glucose, is undoubtedly worse for people with diabetes than sugar. (Sugar is half glucose and half fructose, and fructose does not stimulate insulin release.) It is the phrase "added to the meal plan," and the advice that follows, that is most jarring. To many people it would seem that the ADA is saying that it is okay to make things worse as long as you take more drugs. The "(A)" mark indicates that they consider this advice to be their highest level of evidence. They don't cite that evidence, but it is surely not experimental. While this book was being written, the ADA quietly dropped this passage from their 2013 guidelines,[2] but they have not explicitly stated that it was wrong. It is unknown whether the rank and file of ADA membership ever read the organization's follow-up statements, and if so, whether they thought they were of high quality or simply political statements that no one had time to fight. One of the organization's statements from 2012 reads as follows: "Although brain fuel needs can be met on lower-carbohydrate diets, long-term metabolic effects of very low-carbohydrate diets are unclear."[3]

In fact, the long-term effects of low-carbohydrate diets are clear. Very clear. There are trials spanning one or two years, and internet sites and forums make apparent that low-carbohydrate is a way of life for many people with diabetes. Although personal stories are hard to document, we would have heard if there were any indication of long-term problems. The medical establishment has been obsessed with finding fault with low-carbohydrate diets, and over forty years, they have found nothing. Zero. Zilch. Zip. More important, there is no reason to suggest that there would be any long-term effects. In science, you don't start from scratch. You don't assume that there is harm unless there is a reason to. Nothing about reducing carbohydrate suggests harm. The ADA's use of the word *unclear* implies conflicting data, but there are no conflicting data and there is no reason to expect any. I suggested to a spokesperson for the ADA that the organization was stronger on what they were opposed to than on anything positive they had to offer. She admitted that it was a fair criticism. So, why are they opposed to carbohydrate restriction? The ADA guidelines of 2010 say: "Such diets eliminate many foods that are important sources of energy, fiber, vitamins, and minerals and are important in dietary palatability."[4]

If "care should be taken to avoid excess energy intake," then why would you need carbohydrate as an "an important source of energy?" Diabetes is a severe disease—does anyone think that taking extra vitamins and minerals is as important to a person with diabetes as maintaining healthy blood glucose? There is also a subtle switch from using the word "carbohydrate" to refer to the micronutrient, to using it to mean carbohydrate-containing food. Finally, I would suggest that dietary palatability is not the ADA's area of expertise.

The guidelines from the ADA, as from other health agencies, are supposed to be serious, but, in fact, have the character of an infomercial. Their standards are those of selling a product rather than presenting a scientific case. It seems that we are supposed to just take what they say at face value. The ADA is a private organization, but they receive public support, at least in that they are tax-exempt. Their experts are often federally funded as well. Are they really free to say whatever they want without justification? This is the kernel of the crisis in nutrition. Science is still continuous with common sense. It is not okay at all to, as the ADA says, eat more carbohydrate if "covered with insulin or other glucose-lowering medications." If you can take less medication, that is considered a benefit in every disease I know.

Lipid Chemistry

The second half of the quiz is about lipids. The discussion of what to eat frequently boils down to how much fat one should consume. The medical establishment—including the AHA, ADA, Harvard School of Public

Glycemic Index
Politically Correct Low-Carbohydrate

The original questionnaire given to medical students asked one question about the glycemic index. Intellectually, the glycemic index was an important idea. It followed the same principle as low-carbohydrate diets, and was seemingly of practical value. The intention of the glycemic index was to address the experimental effect of carbohydrate on blood glucose. The glycemic index addresses the old idea, pretty much a dogma when I was in school, that simple sugars would cause a rapid rise in blood glucose, but complex carbohydrate—which at that time still meant polysaccharides (starch)—would not. The idea was questioned at some point, however, and it turns out that when you actually measure the effect of foods on blood glucose, it's not easily predictable—that is, it must be determined experimentally. *Glycemic index* (GI) is precisely defined as the area under the blood glucose time curve during the first two hours after consumption of 50 grams of carbohydrate-containing food. In other words, it is the total amount of blood glucose for a fixed time period after ingestion.

Whatever its promise, low-GI diets have evolved to be a politically correct form of carbohydrate restriction, and it is questionable if they have any value at all. Eric Westman, who has experience with both kinds of diets, put it well: "If low-GI is good, why not no-GI?"

GI is mainly influenced by the absolute concentration of glucose in the food, the extent to which glucose appears in the blood (not necessarily from the food itself), and the quantity of other nutrients such as fat or fiber in the carbohydrate-containing food that might slow the digestion or absorption of carbohydrate. The individual personal variation makes it doubtful that GI diets are useful at all. In comparison to simply reducing carbohydrate, low-GI strategies are complicated and require looking up and calculating values, a feature that might be appealing to some, but is probably annoying to most.

The difference between intensive variables, such as caloric density, and extensive variables, such as total carbohydrate eaten, was brought out at the beginning of the quiz. GI is an intensive variable. Two bowls of cereal have the same GI as one. If there is not much carbohydrate (or really much glucose) in a food, it will have a low GI, but it could still have a large effect if you consume a lot. The glycemic load attempts to correct this problem. The *glycemic load* (GL) is defined as the GI multiplied by the grams of carbohydrate in a sample of a particular food. Obviously, GL is still an intensive variable. You still have to know how much is consumed. More important, are you really sure that GL will really be different from total carbohydrate, which is easier to calculate?

There is also the overall character of using GI. A slice of white bread has a high GI. The GI will go down if you smear a tablespoon of butter on the bread. It will go down still further if you add two tablespoons of butter. If you could somehow butter infinitely, until for all intents and purposes you have pure butter, you would have a GI = 0, which is probably not helpful for those who want to use the GI as a guide to eating.

One final ambiguity: GI measures blood glucose. Fructose, a sugar of great current interest (because it is 50 percent of sucrose and slightly more than 50 percent of high-fructose corn syrup), is partially converted to glucose in two hours, which is why the GI of fructose is 20 and not zero. In fact, more is converted after that time, severely compromising any assertion about the differences in effect of the two sugars. Sucrose has a GI of 70, which is roughly the average of glucose and fructose. Thus, ice cream has a lower GI than potatoes. Yet now we can't recommend ice cream because of the high fructose. Lower GI or lower fructose? How can you do both without saying "low-carbohydrate" out loud? This tangled web is woven out of the failure to face scientific facts. This aspect of the nutritional crisis is probably best addressed by ignoring glycemic index altogether.

Health, and National Institutes of Health (NIH)—has been on an antifat crusade for fifty years. No experiment will make them change their point of view—or more precisely, clearly describe their point of view, which they can apparently mold and reform to fit any challenge. Low-fat products are still everywhere and low-fat is still recommended in one way or another. The diet–heart hypothesis holds that lipid in your diet, particularly saturated fat, will raise one or another lipid fraction in your blood, which will in turn cause you to have a heart attack. They've put it to the test—big, expensive clinical trials with tens of thousands of subjects, hundreds of millions of dollars—and it consistently fails. To figure out what's going on, and to avoid the path to poor health, you have to understand the details. Some of the details involve more chemistry. Many terms in the popular media are used incorrectly and contribute to the current crisis. A little precision will help you understand the problem.

First, you need to know that the term *lipid* refers to a diverse collection of chemical compounds, all of which are sparingly or not at all soluble in water. The group includes fatty acids, fats and oils, cholesterol, and derivatives of these compounds. Directly applicable here are the fats and oils and their constituent components, the fatty acids and glycerol. We'll look at fat structure and the meaning of *saturated* and *unsaturated* fat.

The crux of the crisis is the packaging of lipids into complex units, the lipoproteins (LDL, HDL, and others) that transport cholesterol and fat. These particles are targeted as surrogate markers for cardiovascular risk. As surrogates, they are of limited value. The extent to which they truly indicate risk is controversial. Much of the revolution in nutrition revolves around facing the fact that a surrogate is not the same as actually getting sick. It is still important to be familiar with them, however. They will be part of your lipid workup when you get a clinical lab test.

The big payoff will be wrapping your head around how fat interacts with carbohydrate, and looking ahead, we will try to understand how carbohydrate can be converted to fat, but, to a large extent, fat cannot be converted to glucose. We will want to grasp how it is that we cannot use our fat stores to keep glucose at normal levels and how it is that the amount of dietary carbohydrate might be more important than the amount of dietary fat in determining how much body fat we have. Now, back to the quiz.

7. A good source of monosaturated fat is:
(check all that apply)

	Student response (%)
☐ butter	8
☒ canola oil	22
☐ corn oil	25
☐ flaxseed oil	26
☒ olive oil	58
☒ avocado oil	38
☐ soybean oil	18

You hear the terms *saturated fat* and *polyunsaturated fat* often, but they are not quite precise; only fatty acids can be unsaturated or saturated. All dietary and body fats and oils are triglycerides (TG), or, more correctly triacylglycerols (TAG). The name tells you about the structure: There are three acyl groups (pronounced "ay-seal"). *Acyl* is the adjective form of acid, and the components are fatty acids whose three acyl groups are attached to the compound glycerol. Fats have an *E*-shaped structure. The three arms of the *E* are the fatty acids, and the backbone is the compound glycerol. As shown in figure 2.1, only the fatty acids can be saturated (SFAs) or unsaturated (UFAs). *Saturated fat* simply means that the fat contains a higher proportion of saturated fatty acids. For unsaturated fat and its variations, *mono-* or *poly-*, the chemical bonds that attach the fatty acids to the glycerol are called ester bonds. You only need to know the term *ester* because when the fatty acids are found alone, especially in blood, they are referred to as free fatty acids (FFAs) or—because they are no longer attached to the glycerol part by the ester bonds—nonesterified fatty acids (NEFAs). So FFA and

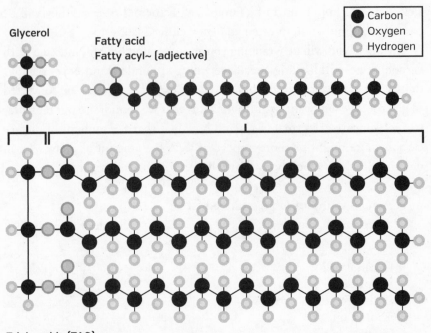

Figure 2.2. Fat structure. Fats and oils are triglycerides (TGs), formally triacylglycerol (TAGs). There are three ester bonds to glycerol.

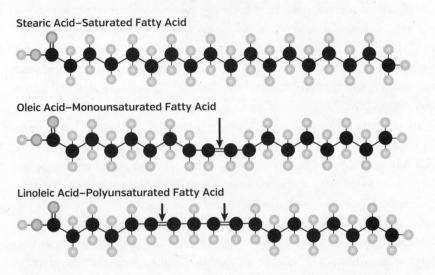

Figure 2.3. Single and double chemical bonds as seen in common fatty acids.

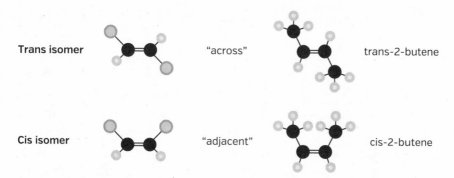

Figure 2.4. Orientation around double chemical bonds. The two carbons in a double bond each have a hydrogen atom and another atom, a carbon, or in the case of fatty acid, a carbon chain. If these are on the same side of the double bond, this constitutes the *cis-* configuration. Otherwise, the bonds are called *trans-*.

NEFA are the same thing. *Fatty acids* are long chains of carbon atoms with a carboxylic acid group. The fatty acids provide the real fuel in fat in the long hydrocarbon chains, much like gasoline. Carbon–carbon double bonds are more chemically reactive and can be converted to single bonds (e.g., with hydrogen atoms, in which case they are called saturated—that is, saturated with hydrogen). *Saturated* means that all the carbon–carbon chemical bonds are single bonds.

Saturated fats, again, have a high percentage of SFAs in the arms of the *E* structure. Similarly, unsaturated fats have high amounts of MUFAs (monounsaturated fatty acids) and PUFAs (polyunsaturated fatty acids). For some fats, however, it is not clear that these terms are useful. One thinks of lard as a kind of pure high-saturated fat, but in fact it is only 41 percent saturated and mostly (47 percent) MUFA, predominantly oleic acid, the main fat in olive oil. From the survey, our students did not have a good sense of what MUFA was. So it is a question of whether you think that lard is half full of SFA or half empty. Most important, as in the epidemiological study described in the introduction, it has been impossible to demonstrate any risk for cardiovascular disease associated with consuming saturated fat—and yet official health agencies continue to insist that there is. If anything, the studies show that carbohydrate is a greater risk than saturated fat, but both correlations are too weak to attribute a significant role to either. I will explore this more as we go along.

The structure of the different kinds of fatty acids are shown in figure 2.3. The major monounsaturated fatty acid is oleic acid. Everybody thinks that monounsaturated fats—those with a high content of MUFA, such as olive oil—are protective of cardiovascular disease, but it is not so clear-cut.

Few fats have only SFAs. Coconut oil is the exception, but those are medium-chain fatty acids (12–16 carbons)—that is, the arms of the *E* in figure 2.3 are shorter than the more common fatty acids. Because of the interest in ketogenic diets, coconut oil has recently become more popular: Medium-chain fatty acids form ketone bodies more readily. In reaction, and presumably because they don't want the public drawing their own conclusions, the American Heart Association has decreed that coconut oil is dangerous, without providing any significant proof of this claim. *Consumer Reports* and the popular media have echoed the AHA's opinions, as if the AHA had come upon a new experimental discovery.

Saturated fats (again, those with a fairly large number of SFAs) tend to be solid, while those with more UFAs tend to be liquid—generally, the more saturation the higher the melting point. To understand why, we need to look deeper into the structure of fatty acids, which brings us to the issue of trans-fats.

Trans-Fats and the Meaning of *Trans*-

When vegetable oils are hydrogenated—the process by which some of the unsaturated fatty acids are turned to saturated—a side reaction can occur that changes the configuration of some of the unsaturated fatty acids from cis- to trans-.

Let me first explain what trans- means, since the nutritional Murphy's Law dictates that confusion will be introduced wherever possible. The carbon–carbon double bond has rigid geometry, so that unlike the single bond, there is no rotation around the bond. Imagine a chain of carbon atoms as in a hydrocarbon such as gasoline or the backbone of a fatty acid. If the bonds are all saturated (single) bonds, then you can think of the molecule as somewhat floppy because of free rotation around the bonds. If there is a double bond in this chain, however, there are two ways to arrange the structure: The two carbons in a double bond can have hydrogen atoms on the same side of the bond (cis-) or on opposite sides (trans-). Figure 2.4 shows the geometry around double bonds.

Almost all naturally occurring fatty acids have the cis- configuration, but it is important to understand that, by itself, this is just a designation for the millions of double bond–containing compounds in the world. Figure 2.3 shows that SFAs have less structure than UFAs, and this lack of structure is why saturated fats tend to be solid: They are easier to pack into a solid. (By analogy, it is easier to pack T-shirts into a box than to pack model Eiffel Towers or heads of Nefertiti.)

MUFAs and the Mediterranean Diet

The Mediterranean diet is widely recommended for its health benefits, but the data are very weak—if there are any at all—and it is not obvious that anybody knows what the diet consists of beyond pouring olive oil on everything. The idea probably originated with Ancel Keys, generally considered the father of lipophobia. Keys originally found a good correlation between fat consumption (actually fat availability) in six different countries and the incidence of heart disease in those countries.[5] It wasn't long, however, before the Secretary of Health in New York State and a professor at Berkeley published a paper showing that there were data from countries other than the six that Keys had studied, which would have significantly weakened the correlation.[6] Keys has generally been characterized as a zealot, although he was probably more open-minded than some of his followers. He was, however, not easily embarrassed and undertook a second study of seven countries.

The Seven Countries Study on dietary availability of fat had an interesting result: The two countries with the highest intake of fat were Finland, which had the highest incidence of CVD, and Crete, which had the lowest.[7] It was deduced that this had to do with the type of fat: saturated in the case of Finland, and unsaturated, in the case of Crete. Things were further complicated when it was later pointed out that there were large differences in CVD between different areas of Finland that had the same diet. This information was ignored by Keys, a pioneer in such approaches to dealing with conflicting data. In any case, the finding immediately led to the recommendations to lower saturated fat, although for most people there was a lingering idea that it was good to reduce fat across the board, despite the lack of correlation in the Seven Countries Study. Subsequently, health agencies were stronger in stepping up the pressure on saturated fat, but not so good at admitting the error in their earlier recommending of low-fat across the board. This is still the state of affairs. The real problem, however, is that even the link between saturated fat and heart disease has been impossible to establish: Direct tests failed immediately and continue to fail. The story of the political triumph of an idea that was clearly contradicted by the science has been told numerous times,[8] and yet the phenomenon still persists. Every time you see a low-fat item in the supermarket, you are looking at an artifact of one of the most bizarre stories in the history of science.

One of the rarely cited responses to the Seven Countries Study was a letter written by researchers at the University of Crete and published in the journal *Public Health Nutrition*.[9] The important part of the letter is this:

> In the December 2004 issue of your journal . . .
> Geoffrey Cannon referred to . . . the fact that Keys and
> his colleagues seemed to have ignored the possibility
> that Greek Orthodox Christian fasting practices could
> have influenced the dietary habits of male Cretans in
> the 1960s. . . . Professor Aravanis confirmed that, in
> the 1960s, *60% of the study participants were fasting
> during the 40 days of Lent*, and strictly followed all
> fasting periods of the church . . . periodic *abstention
> from meat, fish, dairy products, eggs and cheese*, as well
> as abstention from olive oil consumption on certain

Wednesdays and Fridays . . . this was not noted in the study, and *no attempt was made to differentiate between fasters and non-fasters.* In our view this was a remarkable and troublesome omission. (Emphasis added)

The whole sorry tale has now been told many times, most recently and completely by Nina Teicholz in her exposé of the low-fat fiasco, *The Big Fat Surprise.*[10]

Returning to the Composition of Dietary Fat

Going back to figure 2.3, the composition of different dietary fats turns out to be somewhat surprising. It is true that there is a lot of oleic acid (the major monounsaturated fatty acid) in olive oil (73 percent) and canola oil (58 percent). Less well known is that the highest amount is found in avocado oil—and probably most surprising is that oleic acid makes up almost half of the fatty acids in beef tallow and lard (44 percent and 47 percent, respectively). Beef tallow (rendered fat) was what McDonald's used to use to fry their French fries in—at the time, they got the thumbs up from Julia Child—until they were pressured to switch to vegetable oil in a movement spearheaded by Michael Jacobson. Currently the executive director of the Center for Science in the Public Interest, Michael Jacobson might best be described as humorless, uptight, and puritanical. I have been accused of inappropriate behavior in making this characterization, but you can check out his interview with Stephen Colbert for proof (Colbert: "What is the latest thing that you're warning people not to enjoy?") Of course, when McDonald's did switch to vegetable oil, the amount of trans-fat went up, and that got Jacobson riled up again. In any case, most of the saturated fat in beef is stearic acid, which is considered neutral or "heart-healthy," but the question is at least ambiguous—and again, beef fat is only half SFA; the other half is mostly oleic acid, as in the Mediterranean diet.

Canola oil, it turns out, is named for CANadian Oil, Low Acid, an oil isolated from rapeseed (*rape*, from Latin for turnip in this context), which also contains euricic acid. This fatty acid is the star of the 1992 film *Lorenzo's Oil*, but it is not as beneficial as the movie suggests. It is generally considered toxic, and for that reason, it is removed in making canola oil. My original vision of the Quebecoise in their native costumes picking canola fruit from the canola tree turned out not to be correct. There is no canola tree, and the real source, the rapeseed plant, was originally processed to remove the euricic acid.

The rapeseed plant has now been bred to have inherently low euricic acid, and there now really is a plant called canola, the oil of which is one of the major exports from Canada. Processing also produced trans-fatty acids, but this has been removed from current versions of the product.

Back to the quiz. We asked students about the "cholesterol" species that are reported in your lipid profile and that are supposed to be indictors of risk of CVD. What is called cholesterol in this context is actually a supramolecular (more than one type of molecule) known as a lipoprotein, which contains lipid protein.

Lipoproteins: "Good" and "Bad" Cholesterol

There were a few questions from the original quiz that are not reprinted here. Most of our students knew that low-fat diets lower low-density lipoprotein cholesterol (LDL), the so-called "bad cholesterol." LDL is considered bad because it is assumed to correlate well with heart disease, but the correlation is not as strong as many believe. Less than half the people who experience a first heart attack have high cholesterol, and less than half have high LDL (although *high* is, of course, subject to interpretation).

Cholesterol is not a cause of heart disease—we don't know what the cause is—but total cholesterol is considered a very poor risk marker, although it is still treated as a factor associated with incidence of disease. There are, however, better risk markers, including triglycerides and the "good cholesterol," HDL.

8. The diet component that is most likely to
   raise triglycerides (fat in the blood) is: **Student response (%)**

☒ carbohydrate	4
☐ fat	41
☐ protein	19

The phenomenon of carbohydrate-induced hypertriglyceridemia (high blood triglyceride) has been known for at least sixty years. A major contributor is the process of de novo fatty acid synthesis, more usually called de novo lipogenesis (DNL), in which fatty acids are made from other components, mainly carbohydrate. It is significant that the fatty acid that is made in DNL is palmitic acid, the sixteen-carbon saturated fatty acid. Bottom line: Carbohydrate in the diet raises saturated fat in the blood. This was demonstrated most convincingly by experiments at the University of Connecticut[11] described in chapter 7. These experiments revealed that saturated fatty acid in the blood might be harmful, but that its presence is more dependent on the intake of dietary carbohydrate than dietary fat. Our students completely missed the boat on this one.

How much of a risk factor is high triglycerides? Well, it is impossible to tell. The AHA tends to downplay the importance of triglycerides. This is probably related to the need to avoid talking about low-carbohydrate diets, since dietary carbohydrate restriction is the most effective method of reducing high triglycerides except perhaps for total starvation. The AHA has been pretty clear on not endorsing low-carbohydrate diets. On the other hand, triglycerides have clearly become a focus of the ADA, evidenced by their alarmist attitude toward sugar, or fructose in particular. Sugar is carbohydrate, and regardless of whether an increase in fructose is more or less effective than glucose in elevating triglycerides, both will raise triglycerides.

9. In general, what effect does a low-fat diet
   have on HDL-C (high density lipoprotein
   cholesterol, the "good cholesterol")?   Student response (%)

☐ increase	31
☒ decrease	39
☐ no change	30

A low-fat diet reduces cholesterol, both "good" and "bad." The bottom line on the cholesterol problem: The literature tends to show that a subtype of the LDL particle, the smaller LDL, is generally found to be most atherogenic (contributing to a highest risk for CVD). High levels of small, dense LDL are referred to as "pattern B" and this pattern is most dependent on the level of carbohydrate, rather than the level of fat. This critical observation has had little effect on official positions of the AHA or other agencies. It would appear that they don't think LDL size matters, but they have not said exactly why not. The AHA did, however, in 2000, quietly remove their proscription against total fat. You didn't know that?

LDL particle size is not generally measured in a standard lipid profile, and your physician is most likely to look at total cholesterol, or total LDL cholesterol, to determine if you are at risk for heart disease. The recognized surrogate for pattern B is the ratio of triglycerides to HDL. The cutoff is 3.5.[12] If your value is below that mark, you are at limited risk for cardiovascular disease.

It is assumed that the reduction in triglycerides and increase in HDL that is a consequence of a low-carbohydrate diet has a protective effect. As suggested in the introduction, however, it is possible that, outside of well-defined genetic abnormalities, what you eat might have no effect on your risk of heart disease—or, more precisely, individual variations that might predict a link between diet and heart disease have not yet been discovered. We will come back to this theme. The response to doubt separates science from medicine and religion. It is revolutionary to even consider the possibility that the diet–heart hypothesis as it's currently presented is completely wrong. In science, doubt represents an opportunity. In religion, you pray for relief from doubt.

10. The dietary change that is most likely to
    increase the risk of cardiovascular disease is: **Student response (%)**

☐ unsaturated fat → saturated fat	25
☒ unsaturated fat → carbohydrate	28
☐ carbohydrate → unsaturated fat	12
☐ carbohydrate → saturated fat	19
☐ saturated fat → carbohydrate	16
☐ saturated fat → unsaturated fat	0

This is one of the most important observations, because it has been known for so long. I described in the introduction my early research into the literature and my dismay at the results of the Nurses' Health Study,[13] which demonstrated that there was an increase in CVD incidence when fat was replaced by carbohydrate, regardless of the type of fat being replaced. This was astounding given the persistent low-fat message. One would expect that the study, done more than fifteen years ago, would have been the stimulus for a shift away from that low-fat message. That didn't happen.

Assessing the Quiz Results

How did you do? Some critical facts were not known to most of our medical students. In summary, whatever you knew before, the information that you should take forward is this:

- The majority of the increase in calories in the epidemic of obesity and diabetes has been due to a dramatic increase in carbohydrate consumption. The association between the observed behavior of the population in macronutrient consumption and official advice to reduce fat and increase carbohydrates might be causal. How could the advice not have played a role? The bottom line, that reducing carbohydrate is the best treatment for diabetes, suggests that carbohydrate must have played some role in the origins of the epidemic, but this remains unknown. What is established is that the progression of culprits—saturated fat, red meat, white rice—that are "proved" daily by epidemiologic studies to be causes can probably be excluded.
- The crux of the problem in controlling the epidemic of diabetes can be summarized in the following statements:
  - Dietary carbohydrates raise blood glucose in people with diabetes more than other macronutrients.
  - There is no biological requirement for carbohydrate (for anybody).
  - Despite evidence to the contrary, health agencies recommend high carbohydrates (more than 40 percent of total calories).

- The glycemic index and glycemic load are a weak form of low-carb strategy. The logical problems and the limited experimental proof of their efficacy make their use questionable as a primary strategy. They might, however, be of some use, since they still encourage carbohydrate restriction.

- Calories are about processes, not substance, and looking ahead, different processes (oxidation in the calorimeter versus metabolism) make different use of the calories.
- On the technical side: It's good to pay attention to the difference between intensive properties, such as calorie density, and extensive properties, such as total calories. When you hear people say fat is inherently more fattening, you need to know that doesn't mean anything.

The major points about lipids from the second part of the quiz include:

- The terms *saturated* and *unsaturated* can only be applied to fatty acids, the constituents of fats and oils. The composition of common fats and oils is different from popular conceptions (e.g., beef tallow is almost half oleic acid, the main fatty acid of olive oil.)
- The dietary change that has the greatest effect on cardiovascular risk factors is replacement of fat with carbohydrate. Low-fat diets reduce LDL, but low-carbohydrate diets reduce the important subfractions, the pattern B, that are more atherogenic. Reducing carbohydrate also improves HDL. The real question, however, is whether reducing carbohydrate diminishes the actual incidence of CVD. It would be difficult to answer that question, but it must be considered. What you might not have known before the quiz is that our current state of knowledge does not provide evidence that what you eat will make any difference in your risk of heart disease.
- The ambiguity or, more precisely, the near absolute failure of the diet–heart hypothesis contained the seeds of the first low-carb revolution. We'll look at this in the next chapter, and I will explain why another revolution is needed.

CHAPTER 3

The First Low-Carbohydrate Revolution

The first low-carbohydrate revolution dates from about 2002. As is frequently the case in politics, the revolutionaries saw themselves as a loyal opposition and probably didn't think of their ideas as particularly iconoclastic. Dr. Atkins was an established physician who was undoubtedly only trying to help. He was surprised at the vehement backlash. Unfortunately his response to criticism was less like that of John Adams than that of John's cousin, Samuel Adams, who was described in *Don't Know Much About History* as being better at brewing dissent than beer. It is doubtful that much could have been done, though. Like political revolutions, scientific revolutions usually have to be won more than once. Gary Wills described the Gettysburg Address as a statement that the Civil War was a second American Revolution.[1] People of my generation might see the civil rights movement as a third. It's often the same for revolutions in science: We are taught that atomic theory comes from John Dalton, the Manchester schoolteacher who proposed it in 1799, but atoms were not truly accepted as real things, rather than convenient models, until Einstein nailed it in 1905.

The idea that dietary carbohydrate, sugars, and starches have some unique power to make animals fat is very old. It would be hard to identify the first farmer who fattened animals for market by feeding them grain. Brillat-Savarin, the father of modern gourmet cooking, generalized the fattening principle to human beings, and claimed that there were folks who were "carbophores"—in fact, he admitted to being one himself.[2] The mechanism—the anabolic effects of the hormone insulin, stimulated primarily by the sugar glucose—was a well-established physiologic phenomenon before the first low-carbohydrate revolution. The scientific literature provides many examples of weight loss from carbohydrate restriction and links it to something beyond the reduction in calories that usually comes with such a diet. Although it has been around in one form or another for a long time, carbohydrate restriction only became revolutionary with the ascendancy of a kind of low-fat nutritional-medical monarchy, backed by powerful influences.

The first edition of the original Atkins book[3] appeared in the 1970s, right around the time of the codification of low-fat as the desirable diet. The Atkins diet was so vehemently denounced that it gave rise to congressional hearings. An amusing moment occurred when the American Medical Association (AMA) asserted that one of the dangers of a low-carbohydrate diet for weight loss was that it might lead to anorexia. Overall it was an indication of the unwillingness of the medical professions to tolerate dissent.

As in political revolutions, the first low-carbohydrate revolution was stimulated by a kind of manifesto, a document that historians now describe as being a call to action. The equivalent of Thomas Paine's *Common Sense*, which fired everybody up for the American Revolution, was a 2002 article by Gary Taubes in the *New York Times Magazine* titled "What If It's All Been a Big Fat Lie."[4] Later expanded into the book *Good Calories, Bad Calories*,[5] the article documented the political ascendancy of the low-fat paradigm and the establishment of something like the Court of Low-Fat.

The AMA, the AHA, and a number of influential physicians were all received at court. The media and the government, including the McGovern committee, went along with it. Tom Naughton's comedy documentary *Fat Head*[6] includes a clip of McGovern explaining in 1977 that Congress did not have the luxury of waiting for all the science to be in.

The McGovern hearings began a pattern of ignoring dissenting voices, like that of Philip Handler, head of the National Academy of Sciences, who testified that there was little science behind this rush to judgment. I recognized Handler as part of White, Handler, and Smith, the group of authors that wrote one of the few comprehensive biochemistry texts at the time—that is to say, he was a very well-known biochemist.

The Lipophobes and Their Opposition

There were many experimental and clinical trials that set out to prove the diet–heart hypothesis. The first, the Framingham Study, which continues today, is a massive survey of the behavior of residents in this large Massachusetts town. The original results showed no effect of dietary total fat, saturated fat, or cholesterol on CVD. The study did initially find an association between blood cholesterol and CVD, but the correlation wasn't a knockout, and it became weaker as the study continued. This original positive but unsustainable association is now a classic in epidemiology, taught in statistics classes. The fact that diet did not correlate with CVD is less often discussed, and in the later data on cholesterol, some age groups (men, 48–57 years old) actually displayed greater risk with lower cholesterol.

The results of the Framingham Study were buried for years until the statistician Tavia Gordon had them published in 1968, almost ten years after the data had been analyzed. Publication of the data should have been the death of diet–heart hypothesis right there. If fat was as bad as they said, there wouldn't have been a single study that failed to prove it. Not one. In actuality, almost every one of the dozen or so large trials conducted since Framingham has also failed. Science, however, was not the major force behind the denial of evidence. The lipophobes, as Michael Pollan calls them,[7] continued to dismiss each experimental failure as the loss of a minor battle in a war where victory would surely fall to them: just one more big clinical trial, just another hundred million bucks and you will see how bad fat is. Even in 2001, when the AHA removed its proscriptions against total dietary fat, it was done without fanfare. As a result, it is likely that most consumers think that AHA still recommends reduction in overall dietary fat. They're still down on saturated fat, and of course, trans-fat (the latter being a moot issue since it's been almost entirely removed from the food supply), but the truth is that the AHA has given up on total fat.

Although preceded by other exposés, Taubes's *Good Calories, Bad Calories* was the most compelling presentation of how nutritional science had been taken over by lipophobes. Numerous retellings have followed. Nina Teicholz's *The Big Fat Surprise*[8] is of comparable literary quality to *Good Calories, Bad Calories*, and is more explicit in its condemnations of the players. Ultimately, with control over the NIH, the low-fat mafia could now resist all scientific argument and dismiss all of the experimental failures to provide any sort of reasonable case. The ascendancy of low-fat was, and still is, coupled with a special hatred for low-carbohydrate diets and especially for their main exponent, Dr. Atkins, even after his death.

The low-fat idea wasn't good to begin with, but of all the tests of the idea that failed, one after another, nothing was more embarrassing than the Women's Health Initiative (WHI), which reported in 2006: "Over a mean of 8.1 years, a dietary intervention that reduced total fat intake and increased intakes of vegetables, fruits, and grains did not significantly reduce the risk of coronary heart disease (CHD), stroke, or CVD in post-menopausal women." A multicenter, nearly $400 million study, the WHI had assigned 19,541 postmenopausal women to the dietary intervention and had a control group of 29,294 women in a free-living setting. As such, its failure should have been a bombshell.

It was not long before Dr. Elizabeth Nabel, director of the National Heart, Lung, and Blood Institute of the NIH, appeared on television to assure the nation that the recommendations had not changed regardless of the study's findings. You really did still need to reduce saturated fat, she insisted. Nothing's changed, despite the study they funded explicitly showing that change was needed.

The situation was serious. The refusal to accept the failure of a scientific test, and the stubborn insistence on doctrine, caused palpable harm. The WHI women weren't getting any better, and the population at large, doing its best to adhere to low-fat, was getting fatter and more diabetic during this period. Refusal to see the WHI for what it was represented a clear statement that the lipophobe movement, starting at the top at the NIH, was going to stonewall any effort to change.

"The Shot Heard 'Round the World"

If Taubes's "What If It's All Been a Big Fat Lie" was the *Common Sense* of the first low-carbohydrate revolution, then the "shot heard 'round the world" was the report by Gary Foster and coworkers[9] showing that the Atkins diet actually improved markers for cardiovascular disease, the lipophobes' main "concern" about low-carbohydrate diets.

Foster's demonstration had a big impact because he spoke for the whole nutritional establishment. He later described, in public lectures, how he and his collaborators had been having lunch at a scientific meeting, bemoaning their inability to sweep the Atkins diet from their sight. They decided to get a grant to trash the diet, and so they did. One suspects that their intent was clear in the grant application: not to test the efficacy of the Atkins diet—that would've been nearly impossible to fund—but to show just how bad it was. So they carried out a one-year study comparing a low-carbohydrate diet modeled on the Atkins diet with a low-fat diet. What they found, contrary to the conclusion they'd hope for, was that "the low-carbohydrate diet produced a greater weight loss (absolute difference, approximately 4 percent) than did the conventional diet for the first six months."This part was not a surprise even to the authors. Everybody knew somebody who had lost a lot of weight on the Atkins diet, and nutritionists had more or less accepted the idea that low-carbohydrate diets were good for weight loss, though they usually insisted that it was "just a reduction in calories." (If you've tried to lose weight, you know that there is no "just" about it.) The kicker, however, was that Foster reported:

> After three months, no significant differences were found between the groups in *total or low-density lipoprotein cholesterol* concentrations. The increase in *high-density lipoprotein cholesterol* concentrations and the *decrease in triglyceride concentrations* were greater among subjects on the low-carbohydrate diet than among those on the conventional diet throughout most of the study. Both diets significantly decreased diastolic blood pressure and the insulin response to an oral glucose load.[10] (Emphasis added)

In other words, the low-carbohydrate diet was better on HDL ("good cholesterol") and especially on triglycerides. Most importantly, there was no increase in LDL, which is what your doctor uses as the traffic light for determining whether you need to be prescribed statins.

More Work Needs to Be Done

The conclusion of the Foster study: "Longer and larger studies are required to determine the long-term safety and efficacy of low-carbohydrate, high-protein, high-fat diets." This strange conclusion indicates the persistent difficulty in making progress. Low-fat diets do worse on most markers, and are at best a draw on the others, yet we are supposed to be worried about the low-carbohydrate diet? If the low-fat diet is worse, shouldn't we be worried about long-term safety and efficacy of that diet instead? Somehow the conclusion consistently drawn from Foster's experiment was that the "diets were the same at one year"—that it was a draw. There are probably sporting events where the champion keeps the title in the case of a draw, but the idea that the low-fat diet was some kind of champion with a long-term record of success is absurd. The allegedly "prudent" and "moderate" low-fat diet is exactly the one that gave us the epidemic of obesity and diabetes in the first place.

Ad Lib Versus Calorie Restriction

Beyond the obvious bias, Foster's study was compromised in its experimental design. People in the low-fat group were directed to consume an explicitly low-calorie diet: They were required to eat what they were told. In the low-carbohydrate group, on the other hand, participants were allowed to eat anything that they wanted as long as they kept carbohydrates low. (Even if you believe that the diets were actually equal, which diet would you go for?) This protocol was used because Foster et al. were not testing the principle of reducing insulin fluctuations as a means of controlling metabolism. The study was not testing, as in the title, "a low-carbohydrate diet for obesity." Instead it was testing the Atkins diet and perhaps, in the authors' minds, Atkins himself. (After all, the Atkins diet said that you didn't have to count calories—anathema to traditional nutritionists.) The experiment, in reality, was testing two principles: that carbohydrate restriction means greater satiety, allowing you to regulate calories implicitly; and that the Atkins diet, calorie for calorie, is more effective for weight loss. Testing both at once was more demanding than isolating the variables. The low-carbohydrate diet's better results might have been due to either or both principles, but it's impossible to know because of the flawed experimental design.

The dietary protocol was not the only problem. Data were analyzed according to a bizarre method known as intention-to-treat (ITT). In this method, data from the subjects who had dropped out of the study were included in the results by "imputing" values based on previous measurements. The difference between "imputing" and making stuff up is hard to figure out. ITT doesn't make any more sense than you'd think from this brief description, but that's simply how things are (see chapter 16 for a more in-depth discussion). Beyond the obvious lack of common sense, an ITT will always make the better diet look worse than it actually is. In this event, though, those in favor of carbohydrate restriction were sufficiently happy to see the positive outcome, and they were disinclined to be too critical of the methods. At face value, the lipophobes had their shot and they lost. They tried to maintain a façade of impartiality while still putting the burden of proof on low-carbohydrate, but it still didn't help their case. So, what happened to the first low-carbohydrate revolution? Why didn't it move forward? How did low-fat loyalists prevail in the face of such strong scientific evidence?

What Stopped the Revolution?

It was an opportunity. The public had a chance to see if the low-carbohydrate idea would work. Many did try it, and many had great success. Popular articles were written about the phenomenon. Low-carbohydrate wasn't equally effective for everyone, but frequently, it seemed miraculous. People described how the "pounds melted away." So why didn't it move forward? First, there was poor understanding of what actually made the diet work; and second, there was a proliferation of products designed to make low-carbohydrate "easier," because it was perceived, incorrectly for the most part, as a difficult diet strategy. This allowed the company Atkins Nutritionals and other similar ventures to sell a lot of products, many of which were not always helpful. They are still doing that. These products help some dieters stay on track, but their artificial character made them suspicious, and the move toward natural food has made their reputation worse. The low-carbohydrate community itself mostly emphasized low-carbohydrate and, oddly, there was little disappointment when Atkins Nutritionals declared bankruptcy in 2005, though it has since been resurrected and continues to offer substitutes for the carbohydrates that you are giving up. Particularly troubling was the proliferation of products containing sugar alcohols—carbohydrates that are digested slowly, if at all, and were therefore presumed to not contribute to blood glucose. Untested and poorly understood, sugar alcohols gave some people intestinal problems, but more importantly, they cast what should have been a straightforward diet in a slightly bizarre light. Yet in the end, it was not Atkins Nutritionals or any other company, but the nutritionists and the professors of medicine who stopped the first low-carbohydrate revolution. They had a million objections and they got the media on their side.

The Problem with Dietitians

What was remarkable about the whole state of affairs was that the low-fat strategy had failed in competition with a real alternative. Low-fat could not compete with low-carbohydrate, even with the experiment set up in its favor and the authors putting a positive spin on the data. It was a direct challenge to nutritional orthodoxy, but the stalwarts of the old nutritional order did not go gentle into that good night. What torpedoed the first low-carbohydrate revolution were the nutritionists. They had the chance to tell the public, "If you do want to try a low-carbohydrate diet, this is what we recommend." Instead, they acted as if Foster's paper had never existed and they ignored those studies further supporting carbohydrate restriction that followed it.

Nutrition has never been highly thought of. The field derives from the practical job of making institutional menus. The advances of physiology and biochemistry meant that nutrition increasingly overlapped with more solid science, but the field was, and is, very slow to change. Nutritionists have attempted to put on the mantle of professionalism. They are currently trying to establish the newly renamed Academy of Nutrition and Dietetics (AND), and to secure their status as the sole voice on nutrition, with the right to legally repress anybody else. Recently they tried to stop low-carbohydrate proponent Steve Cooksey from "offering counseling" on his blog despite appropriate disclaimers. Thankfully the courts decided that the First Amendment was still the law of the land and left Cooksey's accusers with egg white on their faces. However, the case, now replayed in several similarly ugly conflicts and described in later chapters, highlights the adversarial state of nutritional science and the intolerance of dissent. For those familiar with computer logic and with a taste for computer-nerd humor, my own group may rename itself OR (Objective Research) and plans to refer to the Cooksey affair as NAND-gate.

Underlying all of the resistance is the idea that only long-term, large-scale studies are important, an inaccurate assumption that nutritionists use as a basis for ignoring the smaller studies that are better controlled and provide more information. Small studies are not worse—they are generally better. More important, the quality of a study is not simply determined by the size or length of the study. But once again, the implicit assumption remains that the long-term studies have supported a low-fat diet—a prudent diet, a diet of moderation, a diet with proven success, a diet that can work for all of us. There is no such diet and there never was. The long-term studies have failed, almost every single one: the Framingham Study, the Oslo Diet Heart Study,[11] the Western Electric Study,[12] The Women's Health Initiative,[13] and probably two dozen others. They showed no value in reducing dietary fat or saturated fat for prevention of heart disease or any other health conditions, and in the biggest trial of all, the "full-population trial" of Americans during the obesity epidemic, it was increased carbohydrate, not fat, that was actually harmful.

To be fair to nutritionists, doctors also played a part in the deception. Undeterred by their lack of training or experience in biochemistry or nutrition, it was de rigueur for junior faculty in a department of medicine to write a review trashing the Atkins diet. Some of these critiques even stated that the main flaw of low-carbohydrate diets was their failure to conform to the USDA dietary guidelines and other institutional recommendations. In other words, they faulted a diet whose central premise was that the USDA recommendations were bad, for not conforming to those recommendations. This is a known logical fallacy that was called "begging the question" before the phrase lost its original meaning: using the question as part of the answer.

Failure to Accept Failure

Stepping back and looking at the big picture, the most striking thing was the inability of low-fat diets, even those low-fat diets that did lower cholesterol, to provide a significant impact on cardiovascular outcome, or really, on anything else. Very large, very expensive clinical trials of low-fat dietary strategies failed, and yet our tax dollars continue to pay for similar trials. Even in those cases where we didn't have outcome data about heart attacks

or deaths, and instead had to look at the risk factors—the different cholesterol forms: HDL, LDL, and their subfractions—it turned out that the
effect of reduced fat was at best ambiguous, whereas dietary carbohydrate
typically had the major effect. As carbohydrates were increased, most of the
risk markers got worse. (I should note that these markers and their association with outcome were not sufficient to attribute cause, but that had not
stopped such interpretations when it was low-fat that reduced risk factors.)

If we go beyond the original idea of total blood cholesterol as a major
risk factor (less than half of the people who have a first heart attack have
high cholesterol), and if we instead look at the different forms of the
lipoprotein particles that are actually measured in clinical tests of blood
cholesterol, carbohydrate restriction becomes the "default diet," the one to
try first for general health. It is important to acknowledge, however, that
while low-carbohydrate diets look better for CVD risk factors, we have the
same problem that we have with fat: There is little in the way of evidence
that lowering carbohydrate can actually prevent CVD. Given its success
in treatment of the collection of health markers referred to as metabolic
syndrome, it would be surprising if reducing carbohydrate did not help in
prevention—but at this point, what we know is very little. We are left with
the real possibility that there is nothing at all to the diet–heart hypothesis,
and that diet might not be a major player at all in CVD, except in cases of
well-defined genetic conditions. It's very surprising, given our current view
of things, and it's likely to change as we learn more—but you have to go
with the data.

PART 2

Nutrition and Metabolism

CHAPTER 4

Basic Nutrition

Macronutrients

C arbohydrate, fat, and protein represent the major macronutrients because of the large quantities in which they are consumed. Micronutrients include vitamins and minerals, which are only taken in small amounts. It has become common to refer to foods as either "nutrient-rich" or "nutrient-dense," or not, according to whether they're thought to have high amounts of micronutrients. Some people, including me, are annoyed by this lack of precision. After all, macronutrients are also nutrients, and it would make more sense to say "micronutrient-rich" if that is the intended meaning. Readers should be aware of this lack of precision moving forward.

This chapter describes the primacy of macronutrient composition for metabolic effects. During the years from 1970 to 2000, roughly the period when observers began to notice an obesity epidemic, people consumed an excessive number of calories, the majority of which came from carbohydrates. The total amount of protein, usually the most stable part of the American diet, did not change. Fat, if anything, went down.

The Basics of Carbohydrate Chemistry

Chemically, the class of compounds called carbohydrates includes: simple sugars (monosaccharides), such as glucose and fructose; combinations of two simple sugars (disaccharides), such as sucrose, which is made up of one glucose and one fructose; polymers (polysaccharides), such as starch and glycogen; and derivatives of the sugars (e.g., the so-called sugar alcohols).

Alcohol—that is, ethanol—is not a carbohydrate despite what you might hear on YouTube. Whatever the extent to which sugar can make

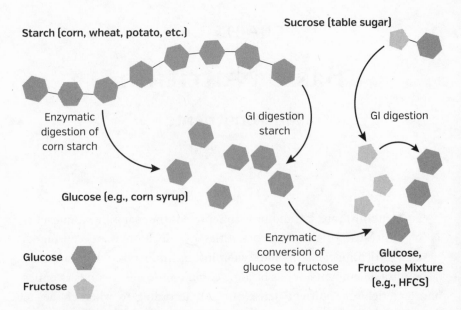

Figure 4.1. Structure and transformations of the common carbohydrates. Starch is a polymer of glucose. In digestion, the glucose units are released and absorbed as such. Sucrose is a dimer of fructose and glucose, and digestion produces the two monosaccharides.

you as loopy as alcohol, the two compounds are simply not the same on a chemical level. A horse is not a dog. One of the reasons that we make Pre-Meds study organic chemistry is in hope that the precision in naming organic compounds will carry over into pharmacology. It is likely that manufacturers started spelling klonopin (an antidepressant) with a *k* because they didn't want physicians to accidentally prescribe clonidine (an antihypertensive).

In terms of formal chemistry, sugars are polyhydroxy aldehydes and ketones. The most common sugar is glucose, and it almost always cyclizes (folds up) in the form of a hexagon, at least in aqueous solutions. Fructose can also form a six-membered ring, but it is more likely to cyclize in a pentagonal shape, as shown in figure 4.1, which provides a simplified representation of the common sugars and related polymers. You can see from the figure that starch is a polymer of glucose (polysaccharide), and that it breaks down into simple sugars during digestion. If you never did the experiment in grade school, you can try chewing a piece of bread for several minutes. The sweetness that develops is the result of digestive enzymes in saliva that catalyze the conversion of the bread's starch into sugar (glucose). Not all starch molecules are as simple as the one depicted in figure 4.1: While some starch molecules, called amylose, do have a linear structure, other types, called amylopectin, have many branch points.

Glycogen: Glucose Savings Account

Glycogen is a highly branched polymer of glucose that serves as the storage and supply depot for body glucose flux. The liver, a kind of command center of metabolism, provides glucose for other organs, and muscle, the main consumer of glucose, stores glycogen for its own use. The liver has the highest concentration of glycogen, but there is more muscle tissue in the body, so it is muscle that possesses the highest total amount of glycogen.

Glycogen is a dynamic storage site. The extensive branching means that there are a lot of ends from which glucose units can be chopped off as needed. It also means that glycogen occupies a lot of space. Children with one of the inborn errors of metabolism known as glycogen storage diseases will have visibly distended abdomens due to the liver increasing in size (hepatomegaly) to accommodate glycogen stores, which in these diseases can no longer be broken down.

We think of glycogen as desirable because of its association with endurance in sporting events. This association is the basis for carbohydrate loading the day before a marathon, but, even in the area of athletics, things are not clear-cut: Marathons are mostly run on fat, even if you are not adapted to a low-carbohydrate diet. Jeff Volek and Steve Phinney have recently trained marathon runners and other elite athletes to perform on very low-carbohydrate ketogenic diets. The athletes do well. They win races, describe perception of greater stamina (not "hitting the wall"), and, surprisingly, they maintain glycogen stores—that is, they run on fat instead of depleting glycogen. It should be noted, however, that a ketogenic diet for athletes depends on a training and accommodation period.

On a low-carbohydrate diet, glycogen storage tends to be reduced, typically by around 60 percent with very low-carbohydrate intake (<100 g/day). However, as I discussed earlier, metabolism does not run on mass action (how much is available) but rather on hormones and enzymes—so under conditions of low-carbohydrate intake, glycogen will be replenished by the glucose produced from gluconeogenesis, thus maintaining storage. It is important to understand that gluconeogenesis and glycogen metabolism are really one process: Glucose synthesized from protein might be stored as glycogen and then only later appear in the blood. An important feature of a carbohydrate-restricted diet, however, is the switch to a metabolic state that runs on fat rather than carbohydrate.

Glucose is at the center of metabolism. Looking ahead to chapter 5, the main theme in human biochemistry is that there are two major fuels: glucose and acetyl-CoA (derived largely from fat and pronounced ASS-a-teel Co-AY). Two fuels and two goals: provide energy and maintain blood glucose at a constant level. Too little blood glucose (hypoglycemia) is not good because some tissues, particularly the brain and central nervous system, require glucose—but too much (hyperglycemia) is also a problem. Glucose is chemically reactive and interacts with several biomolecules through the process of glycation. In the case of protein—the major target—glycation might inhibit biologic activity or may lead to clearance from the cell or circulation. You need glucose, but again, you don't have to ingest any—your liver makes it from protein and other compounds.

A major point that will reappear throughout this book is that carbohydrate and protein can be turned to fat, but while glucose can be made from protein, with few exceptions, you can't make glucose from fat. In the context of the two fuels, this means that glucose can provide acetyl-CoA, but acetyl-CoA cannot be converted to glucose.

Lipid Chemistry: Good Fats, Bad Fats

Most of the fatty acids have common names because they were discovered before we had systematic chemistry and professional panels to set the rules. Some of the names tell you how they were discovered—for example, palmitic acid is found in palm oil, oleic in olives, and caproic and capryllic acids smell like goats (genus *Capra*).

You'll hear a lot of disclaimers about good fats and bad fats, but in one way or another, the government, private agencies, and individual researchers are still recommending that you reduce the total amount fat. The recommendation for reduced fat might be accompanied by an explanation that the type of fat is more important than the total amount, but it usually boils down to some contradictory statement like: "Fat is not bad. Only saturated fat is bad. Eat low-fat foods." The big targets are saturated fat, and of course, trans-fat. The juxtaposition of saturated fat, a natural part of the food chain that has existed throughout human metabolic evolution, and trans-fat, a by-product of industrial modification that was never seen before the twentieth century, is an indication that it is politics, not science, that is at work here. (Note that, as in figure 2.4, *trans-* is a general chemical term, and there are naturally occurring trans-fats that might actually be beneficial. However that is not what is discussed here. As described below, *trans-fats* means the by-product of turning unsaturated oils into solid form.)

The AHA website provides a truly maniacal cartoon video on the hideous Sat and Trans brothers: "They're a charming pair, Sat and Trans. But that doesn't mean they make good friends. Read on to learn how they clog arteries and break hearts—and how to limit your time with them by avoiding the foods they're in."[1]

What's missing from the website is the story behind trans-fat. The crusade against dietary saturated fat, which the AHA and other health agencies fought so vigorously, led to a search for alternatives to butter and lard. It is important to understand that this mission was led by physicians, rather than physiologists or biochemists. Some accused those in charge of trying to carry out a grand experiment with the American people as guinea pigs, but there's no stopping zealots. Butter was seen as the quintessential high-saturated-fat food, and it was clear that no progress could be made without deposing it and installing a substitute.

Wide availability of vegetable oils provided a potential alternative to butter, lard, and other sources of saturated fat. Vegetable oils, however, are liquids, and at least for baking, have to be converted to a more useable form such as margarine or Crisco. You can do this through the process of hydrogenation: Unsaturated oils are "unsaturated" with respect to how much hydrogen is attached to the carbon atoms. Hydrogenation turns some of the unsaturated fatty acids to saturated fatty acids, in effect converting the oil to a solid form. Unsaturated fatty-acid molecules have more rigid structure and are harder to pack into a solid—which is why unsaturated fats tend to be liquid. Converting some of the unsaturated fatty acids into saturated fatty acids made the material more solid and easier to work with. A side reaction in the manufacture of hydrogenated oil, however, is the conversion of some of the oil to the *trans-* form (the names refer to structure).

As you saw in figure 2.4, double (unsaturated) bonds can be *cis-* or *trans-*; most naturally occurring fatty acids are *cis-*, so trans-fatty acids are not normally processed to a great extent. (Note: trans-fats are unsaturated; *cis-* or *trans-* can only refer to unsaturated bonds.) Some biochemists—notably Mary Enig—tried to stop the introduction of products containing trans-fatty acids, but most chemists did not know much about trans-fatty acids and with little support, the low-saturated-fat forces prevailed. At least for a while. When it turned out that trans-fat was the form that correlated best with cardiovascular disease, it was a ready-made scapegoat, and presumably because it was used in so many artificial products, it became the target of health agencies. Of course these groups did not mention that trans-fat in the food supply arose from their own campaign against saturated fat. In the end, trans-fat is a very small part of the diet, and its risk is probably greatly exaggerated. However there is widespread support for its removal among the public, and it is required by law to be removed. Because there's nothing inherently good about trans-fat, nobody wants to defend it.

In contrast to trans-fat, saturated fat has always been part of the human diet and is a normal part of metabolism. Saturated fatty acids are synthesized in your body through a process that is stimulated by a high-carbohydrate diet. This has been known for years. The process is called de novo lipogenesis and is in the biochemistry textbooks, and while it is acknowledged that high dietary carbohydrate led to de novo synthesis of saturated fatty acids, the idea is immediately forgotten when official dietary recommendations are written. So where did we get the idea that fat—and saturated fat, in particular—is unhealthy? Again, the story has been told many times, most succinctly in *The Rise and Fall of Modern Medicine*,[2] most engagingly in *Good Calories Bad Calories*,[3] and *The Big Fat Surprise*,[4] but the death knell for the low-fat idea was, or should have been, the meta-analyses from several groups.[5] A collection of studies, some going back twenty-five years, was not able to find any risk in dietary saturated fat.

The Glucose–Insulin Axis

It remains extremely difficult to eat a zero-carbohydrate diet. It is only very recently that the so-called carnivore diet has become popular. There are no real studies—in the absence of believable or reliable guidelines, self-experimentation is common. Carbohydrate is an inherent part of almost all human diets. There is, however, no biological requirement for carbohydrate in the same way there is for protein, or, to a lesser extent, for fat. Biologically speaking, we've yet to figure out whether differences in carbohydrate type matter, but we do know one simple principle: "High in carbohydrates" is bad advice for people who are overweight and especially for people who have diabetes or metabolic syndrome. For many of them, reducing carbohydrate can constitute a cure—and while we don't know for sure, it is likely that excessive carbohydrate consumption plays a role in how people get fat and diabetic in the first place. We have a grasp on the basic underlying science: Carbohydrate, directly or indirectly, through the hormone insulin, controls the response to other foods. Hormonal systems are very complex but surprisingly, in metabolism, insulin has an overpowering effect. It is an anabolic hormone, meaning it stimulates the buildup of body protein and storage of body material. Insulin is predominant in the storage of nutrients: It encourages the storage of fat and carbohydrate, and increases the synthesis of body protein. Hormones communicate with living cells through the docking proteins known as receptors, and stimulation of the receptors, in turn, triggers the metabolic machinery within the cell.

Carbohydrates, especially glucose, constitute the major stimulus for secretion of insulin. Persistent high-insulin fluxes will bias the body toward storage, and particularly storage of fat. So, even though dietary fat is important, it plays a more passive role than is generally said. The rate at which fat gets stored ultimately depends on the hormones that are present. A high-fat diet with high carbohydrate is very different from a diet with the same amount of fat but lower carbohydrate. Higher carbohydrate, through its effect on insulin, might make the effect of the fat deleterious instead of beneficial. That's the bottom line.

We teach medical students that the flow of dietary fat into stored fat, or into the lipid markers used to characterize cardiovascular risk, is like the flow of water through a faucet. Carbohydrate controls the faucet. If carbohydrate intake is low, the flow stops and fat is oxidized. In the presence of high carbohydrate, on the other hand, insulin increases the rate of fat storage. This is simplified, of course, but not radically so. The main idea, that it is a control problem, not a too-much-stuff problem, is on target.

Diet Comparisons and the Medical Literature

Fat metabolism is only part of the picture. Insulin is a global hormone that regulates carbohydrate and protein metabolism. The evidence for the regulatory function of insulin is there, but not everybody wants to face it. If you confront naysayers, they tell you that the problem is very complex. So, how does it actually play out in the real world? It should be easy to get the answer. Let's consider one experiment that is pretty clear, or at least one that should have been clear: Bonnie Brehm et al. assigned fifty healthy, slightly obese women to an ad lib low-carbohydrate diet or an energy-restricted, low-fat diet, for four months.[6] The results were that the low-carbohydrate women lost significantly more weight.

Brehm et al.'s study yielded both good and bad news. The bad news first: The actual spread of individual values was very large, bigger than what is shown in the paper. Put simply, there are different ways of showing variation in the data, and the method used in Brehm et al.'s paper—the standard error of the mean (SEM)—always makes data look better than they are. The actual spread of values is about four times the size indicated in the publications. So the bad news is that outcomes on the two diets are not highly predictable and from the presentation of the data—group statistics—you can't tell who did what.

The good news is that the big winners must have been the people in the low-carbohydrate group. You don't know if most people in the low-carbohydrate group did better than most people in the low-fat group, or, alternatively, if there were a few really big winners in the low-carbohydrate group that tipped the scale, but you can at least be sure that low-carbohydrate has the possibility of the biggest payoff.

And then there's the really good news: If you read the Methods section, you'll find the experiment followed the same protocols as Foster's famous 2002 study: "One group of dieters was instructed to follow an ad libitum diet. . . . The other group of dieters was instructed to follow an energy-restricted, moderately low-fat diet with a recommended macronutrient distribution of 55% carbohydrate, 15% protein, and 30% fat."

In other words, if you were in the low-fat group, you had to count calories or follow the low-calorie meal plan that they gave you, whereas if you were in the low-carbohydrate group, you could do whatever you wanted as long as you kept carbohydrates low. Even if it's a tie and the results are the same, most of us are going to be happier doing the low-carbohydrate diet since there is no restriction on calories. This is how it was done in the landmark Foster paper and the same pattern has continued since.

As a scientist, you don't always read the Methods section of a paper in great detail unless you are planning to repeat the experiment yourself or there is something unusual in the way the experiment was carried out. If there is something important in the methodology, it should be described in the body of the paper. I admit that when this study was published in 2005, I didn't realize that the standard methodology was a low-calorie diet pitted against an ad lib low-carbohydrate diet. The rationale for this, of course, was that since the Atkins diet did not restrict calories, participants in the low-carbohydrate arm should only be instructed to reduce carbohydrate intake. This might be reasonable from a clinical point of view, but it does make "the diet," rather than carbohydrate—which is easier to control—the independent variable.

Although Brehm et al.'s experiment is far from the best, it is representative of the type of experiment in which the low-carbohydrate diet does better. However, you cannot ignore the big spread in the values. In 2006 a meta-analysis—that is, a reexamination of previous studies—was performed by Alain Nordmann et al. As I'll explain further in chapter 17, meta-analysis is a weak, possibly useless method. The idea is to average previous studies, but most of us agree that averaging errors makes things worse, not better. That said, a meta-analysis usually does give you a chance to see the results from several different studies. The conclusion from Nordmann et al.'s meta-analysis was that low-carbohydrate diets lead to better weight loss. Most of the studies found the low-carbohydrate diet to be more effective at six months but, again, it had no advantage by one year. The reason things got worse after six months is that the experimenters let them get worse: They didn't know how to keep everybody on track. When it's your personal diet, you won't let that happen.

There are now numerous studies that present the same picture. Although the shorter duration studies turn out best for low-carbohydrate, you almost never see a study showing that low-fat is better. Unfortunately, nutritionists tend to consider a draw between the two diets as a win for low-fat, whereas when low-carbohydrate wins, the results are simply ignored, or, as in Foster's study, it's declared that "more work needs to be done." And so we have the recommendations that we do and we are in a current nutritional mess.

A common objection to these studies is that as they depend on diet records—as most do—they are prone to error, and the subjects in the studies often misreport what they eat. Errors in reporting have been documented, but the data are not completely inaccurate—usually they are about 80 percent accurate. All experiments have error, however. It is only a question of how you deal with the error. For inaccuracy in dietary reporting to account for the difference between diets it would be necessary for subjects in the low-fat group to underreport what they ate and for the low-carbohydrate people to overreport what they ate, or both. These errors are certainly possible, but again, from a practical standpoint, it might be good to be on a diet where you think you ate more than you actually did.

Animal Models, Human Subjects

To be fair to the low-fat doctrine, it is easy to be misled. Animal studies are critical in biological science and it seems that mice, especially those bred for laboratory work, will get fat on high-fat diets even without any carbohydrate.[7] How is that possible? People don't usually get fat on high-fat diets, or at least they don't overconsume fat to such a high degree unless their diet is also high in carbohydrate. Mice provide a good model for human metabolism in other cases, too, so this is a serious difference to consider. While carbohydrate is key in human metabolism, the same is not necessarily so in rodent metabolism, where a high-fat diet can bring on obesity, diabetes, and cardiovascular disease even in the absence of carbo-hydrate. We don't yet have a theory to encompass the differences between animal models and human subjects. If our understanding of the catalytic role of insulin is correct, however, then it might well be that mice (who normally live on high-carbohydrate diets) maintain a functionally high level of insulin all the time. In other words, the bias toward an anabolic state that occurs with high-carbohydrate diets in humans might always be "on" in mice.

Whatever the explanation, it's hard for many to recognize that the animal model system we have used so extensively to understand humans might actually have the most impact precisely because *there is a difference* between how people and mice respond to certain treatments. In this case, animal models might offer a clue to human behavior and physiological response through its differences from that of the mice.

The real problem, though, is that we have not faced the results of the practical, experimental tests in humans. We have large, expensive clinical trials with a consistent and reliable outcome: There is no effect of dietary fat on obesity, cardiovascular disease, or just about anything else. The unwillingness to face these failures makes this a remarkable phenomenon in the history of medicine—that it persists in a period of sophisticated science and technology makes it nearly unbelievable. *Unbelievable* is the keyword. One understands that science can be incomplete or might have flaws, but it is hard to understand how the whole establishment could maintain such a misguided opinion on the diet–heart hypothesis. How can they keep doing the same experiment over and over without success? How can they get away with it, and just as importantly, why would they want to get away with it?

In science, excluding a theory is always easier than showing consistency. In this case, if the fat–cholesterol–heart connection was as inescapable a risk as they make it out to be, then none of these big studies should fail. Not one. In fact, almost all fail. Yes, there have been increasing admissions that high-carbohydrate is not a good thing, but these admissions usually come with a qualifier such as "especially refined sugar" or "particularly refined starch," despite the fact that no study has directly compared "refined" and "unrefined" carbohydrates (high-GI and low-GI are not measures of refinement and they are, in any case, weak predictors.) The drastic increase in *total* carbohydrate that has accompanied the obesity epidemic is its most salient feature. Some may choose to ignore it if they don't like it, but it is there.

So, does this mean we can add more fat to our diets, or is fat still bad? It's probably fair to say that most people think that in some way fat it still bad, but the role of fat in the body is itself controlled—directly or indirectly through hormones—by carbohydrate. Deleterious effects of lipid metabolism are ultimately dependent on carbohydrate intake. Perhaps most surprising, the biochemistry shows that although it is the fatty acids in your blood that are the problem, they are more likely to come from dietary carbohydrate than from dietary fat.

Is Carbohydrate Fattening?

I don't understand. I went to this conference and they had a buffet every night, and I really pigged out on roast beef and lobster, but I didn't gain any weight.

—JEFFREY FEINMAN, the author's brother

Nobody manages to avoid weight gain after going on a cruise and pigging out on pasta, but the same isn't true for those, like my brother, who indulge in roast beef and lobster. To return once again to the faucet analogy: Insulin opens the faucet for fat storage but it shuts down the faucet for fat oxidation. At this point, you might ask whether these details matter. Doesn't it all even out in the end? Isn't it just calories in, calories out, or, as they always say in the news releases, "a calorie is a calorie"—and don't the laws of thermodynamics tell us that? It is hard to tell the extent to which you can lose more weight, calorie for calorie, by changing the composition of the diet. One clue, though, is that when experiments show that one macronutrient is less efficient than another (wastes calories as heat), it is usually the low-carbohydrate arm that is less fattening. Critics say that these results are due to inaccurate reporting of food intake, and that it is always just a matter of total calories consumed. Low-carbohydrate diets, they claim, simply reduce total energy intake. It's true that food frequency records can have substantial error, as in the Brehm study. If reduced calorie intake is indeed why the low-carbohydrate group always wins in these face-offs, then as we know, low-carbohydrate participants would have to be overreporting what they ate or low-fat comparisons groups would have to be underreporting what they ate, or both. Wouldn't this be a positive point for low-carbohydrate though? There might be a real benefit to being on a diet where you think you ate more than you did. After all, there is no "just" about reducing calories.

The other hole in the critics' argument is that thermodynamics does not predict that "a calorie is a calorie." Most people who quote the "laws of thermodynamics" (they usually mean just the first law) have never studied thermodynamics. The essential feature of thermodynamics rests not with the first law, which is about energy conservation, but rather with the second law, which says that all (real) processes are inefficient. Energy is dissipated. The variable efficiency (the extent to which energy is wasted as heat) of fat, protein, and carbohydrate is well known, but in the medical literature, it is ignored at will. In cases where total calories turn out to be the controlling variable, independent of macronutrient composition, it is because of the homeostatic (stabilizing) mechanisms of biological systems, not because of thermodynamics. Thermodynamics is my special interest, and we'll come back to the subject in chapter 9.

"The Atkins Diet Is a High-Calorie Starvation Diet"

This quotation is from George Cahill, one of the pioneers in the study of metabolism and the response to starvation. The idea is that the reduction in blood glucose and insulin and the increase in glucagon that accompany lower carbohydrate intake resemble the changes that are associated with total reduction in calories. In starvation, insulin goes down, glucagon goes up, fat oxidation increases, and—at some point— ketone bodies are generated.

In 1992, Klein and Wolfe carried out a defining experiment.[8] The subjects went without food for three days, were given a period of rest, and then went through another three days of starvation. During the second stretch without food, however, the subjects received intravenous injection of a lipid emulsion (fat) that was designed to meet their resting energy requirements. The first period represented a model of early starvation, and the second represented an absence of food intake with adequate energy. Klein and Wolfe measured several physiologic parameters during each period, and as shown in table 4.1, there was not a great difference between the two periods despite the very large discrepancy in energy intake. The levels of free fatty acids were expected to be different—in the first period, breakdown of body fat was required for energy, so free fatty acids would be high; and in the second period, free fatty acids would be lower since injected lipid would be used for energy—but, in fact, the values were the

Table 4.1. Similarity of Starvation and Carbohydrate Restriction

	Free fatty acids (μmol/l)	Fat oxidation (μmol/kg/min)	Glucose (mg/dl)	β-Hydroxybutyrate (mM)
84-hour fast	.92	1.94	68	2.56
84-hour fast + lipid	1.02	1.67	66	2.54

Source: S. Klein and R. R. Wolf, "Carbohydrate restriction regulates the adaptive response to fasting," *American Journal of Physiology* 262, no. 5 (1992): E631–636.

same. Similarly, ketone bodies, which reflect the absence of calories, were reasonably high in the fasting group, but in the second case, with adequate energy, one might have expected low ketone bodies. The explanation of the experiment is that the controlling factor was the level of insulin and glucose. The study concluded that "these results demonstrate that restriction of dietary carbohydrate, not the general absence of energy intake itself, is responsible for initiation of the metabolic response to short-term fasting." The statement is undoubtedly something of an exaggeration—there are other factors that might have modified the results—but the experiment brings out one of the major themes in diet and metabolism: Carbohydrate is a controlling element, whereas dietary fat plays a relatively passive role. Circulating fat, body fat, and fatty acids do play a role in metabolism, but it is wrong to assume that dietary fat equates to body lipids. This is a major theme in this book: "You are what you eat" is not a good principle.

Looking Back, Are Carbohydrates Fattening?

Harper's Illustrated Biochemistry is one of the standard texts in medical and graduate schools. Now in its twenty-ninth edition, it is a multi-authored comprehensive view of the field. I am grateful to Adele Hite of the University of North Carolina for pointing out that in the eighth edition of the text, published in 1961 when it was called *Review of Physiological Chemistry* and Harper himself was the sole author, the close connection between carbohydrate and fat was evident. The chapter on metabolism of carbohydrate began as follows: "In the average diet carbohydrate compromises more than half of the total caloric intake. However, only a limited

Going Without Food

Human metabolism has two goals: to provide energy and to maintain blood glucose at a relatively constant level. In the eight hours or so after a meal—the fed state, or what nutritionists call the postprandial state—diet can provide a greater or lesser amount of the material needed to meet these two needs. If you go long enough without eating, food no longer provides material for metabolism directly—this is referred to as fasting, or the postabsorptive state. When you wake up in the morning after an overnight fast, insulin is low and glucagon is high, so fat is broken down through the process of lipolysis into fatty acids and glycerol (lipolysis is inhibited by insulin and stimulated by glucagon.) The fatty acids are oxidized for energy, and blood glucose is maintained by the processing of liver glycogen. Muscle also stores glycogen that can be broken down. This glucose is used by the muscle itself and is not exported. In simpler terms, as noted before, we can think of muscle as a consumer of glucose and the liver as a supplier, or more generally, as a command center for metabolism.

Gluconeogenesis

Gluconeogenesis is frequently described as a last-ditch source of energy when food isn't available and glycogen is depleted, but in fact, gluconeogenesis is happening all the time. When you wake up in the morning, more than half of the free glucose in the blood or produced from previously stored glycogen comes from gluconeogenesis. Although there is no form of protein formally defined as a storage site, as there is for stored fat or glycogen, muscle can be thought of as providing an internal source of protein, a source that must be replenished from the diet, a dynamic store of amino acids for metabolism.

Is Starvation a Good Way to Lose Weight?
In the fasting state, adipocytes (fat cells) supply fatty acids from
the breakdown of fat. Most tissues, including the heart, oxidize
the fatty acids for energy. Some tissues—primarily the brain and
central nervous system—require glucose, which can be provided
by the combination of glycogen breakdown and replenishment
from gluconeogenesis. The two goals of metabolism are thus
taken care of. Is starvation a good way to lose weight? Of course
it is not. The requirement for amino acids from protein for the
maintenance of blood glucose is the problem. In the absence of
dietary protein, your body will turn to its own sources. Fasting
has become popular, but the breakdown of protein after a day or
two might have physiologic consequences. The answer is not in,
so I would be cautious of a fast for more than twenty-four hours.

amount of this dietary carbohydrate can be stored as such. It is now known
that the un-stored portion of the ingested carbohydrate is converted to fat
by the metabolic processes of lipogenesis."[9]

In other words, the third sentence of the carbohydrate section of a
biochemistry text emphasized the closeness of carbohydrate and fat. In the
twentieth edition (1985), the chapter, now written by Peter Mayes, begins
similarly and continues: "It is possible that in humans the frequency of
taking meals and the extent to which carbohydrates are converted to fat
could have a bearing on disease states such as atherosclerosis, obesity and
diabetes mellitus."[10]

In the current edition, the process of conversion of carbohydrate to fat
now has a chapter of its own. The process is known as de novo lipogenesis,
new synthesis of fat, or more precisely de novo fatty-acid synthesis, since
the immediate product is a fatty acid, the saturated fatty acid palmitic acid
(C16:0). De novo lipogenesis appears to be the explanation of the counterintuitive result, demonstrated in several studies, that dietary carbohydrate
leads to increases in saturated fatty acids in the blood. Chapter 9 describes

an experiment from Jeff Volek, then at the University of Connecticut, where such an increase in saturated fatty acids was greater in the blood of people on a high-carbohydrate diet compared to those on a low-carbohydrate diet, even though the latter had three times the amount of dietary saturated fat.

What About Protein?

In some classes that I teach, I ask the students for the definition of life. I get different answers but I usually say "No, a one-word definition." I try not to drag it out too long or to overact, but the answer that I am looking for is "protein." Everything that goes on in life is controlled by protein, either as the actual component or as the source for other things. Because of its multiple roles in biology and the far more complicated chemistry, I will present here only broad outlines in the context of an answer to an email.

I received the following question:

If one is on a very-low-carbohydrate/high-fat diet, what happens to excess protein that is not needed for muscle repair and growth, and gluconeogenesis? I see two alternatives:

1. It's excreted
2. More glucose is created.

Number 2 seems so unreasonable to me. Would your metabolism actually make more than the little bit it needs? I'm open to a number 3 that I might be too unimaginative to think of. I'm interested in the theory. This isn't a request for diet advice. I like to understand things at the cellular level.

The answer is that it depends on what else is going on, but protein, per se, is not excreted (in the absence of some disease). Protein is a polymer. Unlike glycogen, which is a homopolymer of identical glucose units, the individual units, amino acids, are picked from about twenty different choices. In digestion, protein is broken down to individual amino acids, which are absorbed and reassembled into body protein. The sequence of amino acids defines the biologic function, and this sequence is encoded in the genetic material. The genetic code is largely the code of amino acid sequences.

After digestion and absorption, some of the amino acids that are not used for protein synthesis may be trashed. The nitrogen is converted to ammonia. Ammonia is converted to the compound urea and excreted. The remaining carbon skeleton can be used for energy either directly in the citric acid (TCA) cycle or by conversion to ketone bodies, especially on a very low-carbohydrate diet. Some amino acids can be converted to glucose. Much more than a little bit is needed. The carbon skeleton from amino acids, directly or indirectly, can be converted to fat. So a practical answer is that "excess" protein is recycled: used for energy or for synthesis of glucose.

Protein, as such, is not normally excreted. Proteinuria is an indication of some abnormality, kidney malfunction, or other disease-related nephropathy. Amino acids are excreted at some low level. High excretion of particular amino acids is usually an indication of some metabolic disturbance or inborn error of metabolism. It is important to understand that everything that goes on in the body is mediated by proteins, which turn over all the time, and whereas muscle "repair and growth" is important, it is not the only thing. Body proteins, unlike glycogen or other homopolymers, have specific amino acid sequences and so require a particular makeup. Some amino acids are interconverted and some (essential amino acids) are required from diet.

Current tendencies are to try to encourage vegetarianism or, at least, to encourage reduction of meat consumption. Whatever the moral or practical arguments are, the scientific case is highly questionable. The proliferating studies trying to demonstrate an association between meat consumption and one disease or another are largely bogus, and a couple of these studies are deconstructed in chapter 14. The past few years have also seen a proliferation of "experts" whose training and expertise in nutrition were still being questioned and who have now become authorities on global warming and sustainability of life itself.

CHAPTER 5

An Introduction to Metabolism

T he nineteenth century was a period of political, intellectual, and scientific revolution. Although the politics made more noise, there might be greater long-term impact from the turnarounds in intellectual and scientific fields. Paris in the summer of 1848 was the site of yet another French Revolution. People had taken to the streets and were building barricades just as in *Les Mis*. There was dissatisfaction over rights of assembly and the autocratic government, but rising food prices were perhaps the larger driving force. Whatever the origin of the disorder, faculty at the Collège de France complained that it had "slackened the zeal for research among all of the chemists," and that their time was "absorbed by politics."[1] The intellectual revolution at the Collège, however, was unfolding in Claude Bernard's laboratory.

Bernard, generally considered the father of modern physiology, had been studying digestion in dogs. He found sugar in a dog that he had been dissecting, despite the fact that the animal had not been fed any sugar. The finding was revolutionary because it was generally assumed at the time that any sugar in an animal had to have come from the diet. Furthermore, it was expected that even if an animal had consumed sugar, that sugar would, in the end, be destroyed by oxidation. Antoine Lavoisier had shown more than one hundred years before that animals eat sugar—or any food—for energy, and that the energy comes from oxidation of the food, just as if you were burning food in a furnace. So how did sugar wind up undigested in the animal? Bernard's first thought was that there might be something wrong with the reagent that he had used to detect the sugar, but the reagent was okay—the dog really was making its own sugar. In fact, he soon found that if he fed a dog only meat, there was as much sugar in that animal as there was in another dog that had been fed "sugary soup." Strange as it seemed, he concluded that the dog must have been making its own sugar.

The Discovery of Glycogen and Gluconeogenesis

Although Bernard's experimental findings were occasionally at fault and at times influenced by preconceptions . . . his strength appears to lie in his ability to discard a theory once its experimental basis had been undermined. Even though he was apt not to state frankly that he had been wrong, he nevertheless did change his ideas.

—F. G. Young[2]

It took some further work to show that the sugar was actually being produced in the dog's liver, but by 1857, Claude Bernard had isolated the *matière glycogene*—that is, glycogen. We know now that glycogen is a storage form of carbohydrate, a polymer of glucose. It is actually made from glucose, although the glucose that goes into glycogen may come from something else.

As I explained in chapter 4, glycogen is a highly branched, highly structured polymer, and it is the key player in maintaining blood glucose at a constant level. When cells use up the available glucose, the liver breaks down glycogen to reestablish a constant level. Bernard emphasized this role of glycogen as a supplier, providing glucose to the circulation, but he was not quite right about how glycogen formed in the first place. He knew that glycogen didn't come from fat, and he found through further experimentation that dietary protein seemed to raise glycogen levels even more than dietary sugar (he used fibrin, the blood coagulation protein for his tests). The picture that evolved was that protein was the source of glycogen, which, in turn, could produce glucose. This was not exactly right—if carbohydrate intake is high, ingested sugar is converted to glycogen—but Bernard had discovered something critical: the need for a process that converted other things into glucose, a process now known as gluconeogenesis that would not be fully understood for another hundred years.

Our current understanding focuses on glycogen synthesis and breakdown as a control point in metabolism. Sugar in the diet or in the circulation can be stored in glycogen and then made available when needed. However, it is not only dietary glucose that shows up in glycogen. Bernard was right that sugar could be made in the liver from protein—that is, amino acids from proteins. The glucose synthesized in gluconeogenesis can be exported to the blood, or alternatively, can be used to replenish previously used glycogen, and the new glucose molecules might only appear in the blood at a later time.

Although Bernard understood that glucose came from glycogen, he did not realize that glycogen could also be made from ingested sugar. The key mistake was Bernard's inability to grasp that glucose is present in the blood all the time and it is maintained at a constant level. He didn't get it because he had actually made an experimental error. A lucky one, it turns out.

Sometimes We Luck Out

Bernard's reason for believing that glycogen was not made from glucose came from his measurements of the inputs to and outputs from the liver. Bernard determined the amount of sugar in the portal vein, which brings blood from the digestive tract to the liver (it's not a true vein), and he also measured the amount of glucose leaving the liver in the hepatic veins. His original observations showed that there was little or no glucose in the inputs from the portal vein, but that there was sugar in the hepatic veins leaving the liver. In other words, he could see glucose exiting the liver but no glucose coming in. This observation pretty much made his case that the liver was a sugar-producing organ and that glycogen was being made from something else.

Some of Bernard's scientific rivals said that he was wrong, claiming that they had been able to detect sugar coming into the liver in the portal vein. They were right, of course—we know that there is sugar throughout the circulation and that glycogen is assembled from blood glucose. Bernard had made the mistake of letting some of his preparations sit around too long while the sugar in the portal vein to the liver was being metabolized. Bernard was right to an extent: Usually, more sugar is leaving the liver than is coming in (the liver *does* produce glucose), but the differences are small and the instruments available to Bernard might not have allowed him to detect them. It was this error that allowed him to piece together a picture of a more complicated part of metabolism. Although he got things slightly wrong and had to modify his ideas later, the error allowed him to identify glycogen and to generate the idea of gluconeogenesis. Sometimes we luck out.

Today, we emphasize the need to keep blood glucose constant. We understand that almost all cells in the body can use glucose as an energy source, so having too little is not good. However, it turns out that too much is also not good, because glucose will react with proteins in the blood and tissues to form what are called advanced glycation end-products, or AGEs. These modified proteins can be a factor in aging and degenerative disease. In the popular press and on social media, the negative effects of high glucose have led to the idea that glucose is a toxin, which is surely exaggerated, or at least a mischaracterization of the AGEs.

An Evolving Understanding of Metabolism

Through the work of Bernard and others—particularly Louis Pasteur—the end of the nineteenth century saw the evolution of a science of metabolism, allowing greater understanding of the inner workings of the body and how sources of energy are used. By that point, we knew that blood glucose came from the liver as well as from the diet, and that dietary glucose came from sugars and starches.

Looking ahead, under conditions where there is no food or there is low dietary carbohydrate, there will be a continuing drain on body protein. In the latter case, protein for the body can be supplied from the diet, but ketone bodies provide an alternative source of energy to reduce the dependence on protein. Ketone body synthesis and utilization interact, as one would expect, with glycogen metabolism.

To put this in context, the next section will provide an overview of energy metabolism, illustrating the principle that, in metabolism, there are two goals and two fuels.

The Black Box of Life

Metabolism—the conversion of food to energy and cell materials—is as complicated as you would expect, but it is possible to get an idea of the big picture. The approach here is called the "black box" strategy: getting

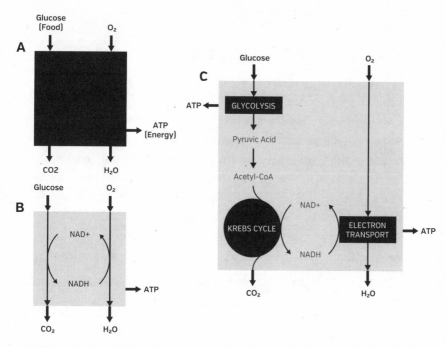

Figure 5.1. The black box approach to metabolism. *A,* The black box of life summarizes how we eat food, take in oxygen, and excrete CO_2 and water. *B,* Inside the black box, we see the oxidation of food is carried out by an intermediate coenzyme NAD+. The product reduces oxygen to water. *C,* The main process. The big players.

as much information as possible by looking at the inputs and outputs of a system without necessarily knowing the details of what's going on inside. As we uncover more details, we can nest black boxes inside each other, thereby organizing the limited information we have. This method is favored by engineers, who are the people most unhappy with the idea that they don't know anything at all.

You likely already have a basic idea of what we do in metabolism: We take in food and oxygen, and put out CO_2 and water. Looking at the inputs and outputs (see figure 5.1), even without knowing a great deal about chemistry, you can figure out that oxidation is occurring within the box—like the burning of fuel to generate heat or run a machine. Technically speaking, it is an oxidation-reduction reaction (redox, for short). Oxidation, in this context, means combination with oxygen. In metabolism, it is frequently the hydrogen atom attached to a metabolite that is oxidized (to water).

Chemical Energy

In physics, energy refers to the ability to do work. As complicated as systems can get, we are basically talking about lifting a weight on a pulley. In chemistry, energy is identified with the progress of a reaction. If a chemical reaction proceeds by itself, at any speed, without the addition of work, we know that we can use it to lift a weight. If you have studied any chemistry, you will remember the equilibrium constant, which tells you how much product you have at the end of the reaction. If the constant is favorable—that is, if you have a lot of product—then the reaction is said to be exergonic, downhill and spontaneous. You can get energy from it.

There are two parts to an oxidation-reduction reaction. In the oxidation of a hydrogen atom (alone or in a compound), the oxygen is said to be reduced. The generalization used in biochemistry is that a compound gets oxidized if it combines with oxygen, and becomes reduced if it combines with hydrogen. (Redox reactions are a fundamental part of all chemistry and the concepts have been highly developed, but this simplification works well in biochemistry.) Like combustion reactions, redox reactions produce energy that can then be used to do work. Some energy is used for mechanical work—moving muscles—but most goes toward chemical work: making body material, keeping biological structures intact, generally keeping things running.

The Two Goals

To review, there are two major goals in human metabolism: first, provide energy for life processes, and second, maintain more or less constant levels of blood glucose. Too little glucose is not good because it is a major fuel, but too much is also harmful because it will react with proteins to create AGEs, as described earlier in this chapter.

Energy in biochemistry is described in terms of a particular chemical reaction. When you study biochemistry, you first examine what the compounds do precisely, but then you use them as abbreviations. Phosphate ion (unattached to other atoms) is abbreviated Pi, where the "i" stands for "inorganic." Although it is now considered somewhat archaic, Pi is still sometimes read as "inorganic phosphate." So, the big energy system in biology is:

$$ADP + Pi \rightleftharpoons ATP + H_2O \quad (1)$$

Energy storage occurs in living systems through the synthesis of ATP from ADP (the other reactants are assumed). In metabolism, you need "energy" from food to make ATP from ADP. Then, when ATP is converted back to the low-energy form, ADP, through hydrolysis (adding water)—that is, when the above equation moves from right to left—energy is released. This energy can be used to do chemical work, and make proteins, DNA, and other metabolites and cell material. The reaction is favored in the reverse direction: It tends toward the release of energy.

Textbooks frequently refer to ATP as a "high-energy molecule," but it is the reaction (synthesis and hydrolysis), rather than the compound itself, that is high energy. For the moment, we can think of ATP as the "coin of energy exchange in metabolism" and the ATP to ADP ratio as the energy state of the system.

The Two Fuels

In order to fulfill the two goals, two kinds of fuels are used: glucose itself and the two-carbon compound acetyl-coenzyme A (abbreviated acetyl-CoA or acetyl-SCoA). Coenzyme A is a complicated molecule, but it's not important to know the details for our purposes. Coenzymes are small molecules that take part in the metabolic changes in living systems. They can be involved in energy metabolism (such as ATP to ADP) or other reactions. The oxidation-reduction coenzymes are the NAD (nicotinamide adenine dinucleotide) molecules, of which there are two forms: oxidized, NAD+, and reduced, NADH.

Most ATP in the cell comes from the oxidation of acetyl-CoA, but glucose can be converted to acetyl-CoA. Acetyl-CoA also comes from fat, and to a smaller extent, from protein. Glucose itself can be formed from protein but not from acetyl-CoA. The significance of this, as we have said, is that fat can be formed from glucose, but with a few minor exceptions, glucose cannot be formed from fat. Historically, the challenge for biochemistry has been to explain how the energy from an oxidation-reduction reaction could be used to carry out the synthesis of ATP, which has a different mechanism (phosphate transfer). The process is called oxidative phosphorylation and was only figured out about fifty years ago.

Breaking into the black box, oxidation of food is separated into two different processes. The food never sees the oxygen but instead there is an intermediary player. The intermediate agent, the redox coenzyme NAD+, does the oxidation of food, and the NADH (the product, the reduced form) is re-oxidized by molecular oxygen. Why do we do it this way? In general, biochemical reactions proceed in small steps to allow for control and for capturing energy. Even if we could do it all in one big blast, like an automobile engine, living tissues do not do well with explosive, high-temperature reactions—we would have little control over them and we would not be able to capture the energy in a usable chemical form.

Glycolysis

Glucose is at the center of metabolism. Glycolysis, the collection of early steps in its processing, is common to almost all organisms. Glycolysis (sugar splitting) ultimately provides two molecules of the three-carbon compound known as pyruvic acid (pyruvate). In most cells, the pyruvate from glycolysis is oxidized to acetyl-CoA, which is the input for aerobic (oxygen-based) metabolism and the main source of energy for most mammalian cells. One of the functions of glycolysis is to prepare glucose for oxidative metabolism—that is, to provide acetyl-CoA. Some cells, however, can run on glycolysis alone. Such cells are said to have a glycolytic metabolism and can convert pyruvate to a number of different compounds, most commonly lactic acid.

Many microorganisms are glycolytic, and much of our understanding of glycolysis comes from the study of bacteria and the process of fermentation. The final product of glycolysis can be very different from one organism to another. Alcoholic fermentation involves the conversion of pyruvate to a two-carbon compound acetaldehyde, which in turn is converted to ethanol. (When you ingest alcohol, your liver runs this reaction backward, converting alcohol to acetaldehyde and then to acetyl-CoA, which is further oxidized.) Other kinds of glycolytic bacteria, like those in yogurt, convert pyruvate to lactic acid (lactate), accounting for the acidity of yogurt. Mammalian cells can also carry out this transformation. The brain, central nervous system, red blood cells, and rapidly exercising muscle are the most common of the glycolytic tissues that produce lactate. It was once believed that the lactate produced by exercising muscle was the cause of delayed-onset muscle soreness (DOMS), but this is not true. Although the cause of DOMS is not known, the lactic acid is metabolized and long gone by the time soreness sets in.

Oxidative Metabolism

Acetyl-CoA is the main substrate for the oxidative process that produces CO_2, which is then released from the black box of life. This process is frequently called the Krebs cycle, after Sir Hans Krebs, who was the pioneer in assembling a coherent mechanism from the various observations of where particular carbon atoms went when different foods were fed to a tissue or organism. Oxidation of such a small molecule as acetyl-CoA would have to take place in a small number of steps, and would not allow the kind of control that it is necessary to keep a biological system responsive to different conditions, so the two carbons of acetyl-CoA are attached to a carrier to form a six-carbon molecule, called citric acid, or citrate. For this reason the cycle is frequently referred to as the citric acid cycle. Complicating things further, citric acid is a tricarboxylic acid, or TCA for short, so the process might also be called the TCA cycle. All three names are used: the Krebs cycle, the citric acid cycle, and the TCA cycle. Krebs himself called it the TCA cycle, so we will try to stick with that.

The TCA cycle is complicated, but I will try to provide a rough description: The substrate, acetyl-CoA, is bound to a carrier to form a compound, citric acid, that is oxidized, stepwise, primarily by the redox coenzyme NAD+. The products of the reaction are CO_2 and the reduced form of the coenzyme, NADH. NADH is the ultimate reducing agent (transfers H) that turns oxygen to water. This process, the electron transport chain, is a

Sources of Acetyl-CoA

Glycolysis is not the only source of acetyl-CoA for the oxidative metabolism of glucose. The major source, for many cells, is fatty acids from fat. The process of converting fatty acids is called β-oxidation. The long-chain fatty acids are chopped two at a time from the carboxyl end. It uses the Greek character β because the break is at the second carbon in the fatty acid chain.

sequence of reactions that, in effect, transfers electrons. The net effect is the reduction of molecular oxygen to water. Somehow this converts ADP to ATP. This is the mechanism for channeling the energy of burning food into the conversion of ATP back to ADP—that is, the storing of chemical energy. The process, still mysterious when I was in graduate school, is now understood. The idea behind it is called the chemiosmotic theory—really no longer a theory—which was largely the work of a single man, Peter Mitchell. It would be a major digression to delve into the overall process here, but I recommend doing some research into both chemiosmotic theory and Peter Mitchell himself. Because it involves oxygen, obtaining energy from the TCA cycle electron transport chain is referred to as oxidative metabolism, distinct from glycolytic metabolism, which might precede it. Glycolysis provides acetyl-CoA for the TCA cycle. Looking ahead, a major feature of cancer cells, referred to as the Warburg effect, appears to be a greater reliance on glycolysis rather than oxidative metabolism, in comparison to normal cells, even when oxygen is present. Explaining the Warburg effect is a major focus of current cancer research.

Ketone Bodies

Ketone bodies have evolved as an alternative energy source under conditions of starvation or carbohydrate restriction. Synthesis and utilization of ketone bodies provide a way of dealing with the biochemical principle stated so many times throughout this book: You can make fat from glucose but you cannot make glucose from fat. None of the energy stored in the form of fat will help in providing glucose for the brain and the central nervous system (CNS). In the absence of dietary carbohydrate or total calories, protein becomes the main source of carbons for gluconeogenesis—and the risk here is that you will break down essential body protein to meet this second goal of metabolism, maintaining blood glucose.

Created in the liver from acetyl-CoA, the ketone bodies, β-hydroxybutyrate and acetoacetate, are four-carbon compounds. They provide a way for acetyl-CoA units (from fat) to be transported from the liver to other tissues, where they are turned back into acetyl-CoA and used for energy. Through this process, protein no longer has to bear the full pressure of providing glucose under extreme conditions.

The brain and CNS cannot use fatty acids for fuel. These and some other tissues are dependent on glucose, at least under normal well-fed conditions. The dilemma in a starvation state, or on a low-carbohydrate diet, is how to supply energy to these tissues. Because you cannot make glucose from fat, amino acids from protein must supply glucose via gluconeogenesis. In starvation, that protein must come from muscle and other body proteins. It is the demand for glucose, rather than total energy, that is the problem under extreme conditions. (On a low-carbohydrate diet, the problem is avoided because of the availability of dietary protein. While low-carbohydrate diets are not necessarily high in protein, a somewhat higher level is needed to supply material for gluconeogenesis.)

The ketone bodies are derived from fatty acids, but unlike fatty acids themselves, they can be used by the brain and CNS because they supply acetyl-CoA directly. The evolutionary advantage of ketone bodies is that they provide a way to avoid the breakdown of body muscle stores. For this reason, ketosis (ketone bodies in the blood) is generally described as "protein-sparing." In the beginning stages of ketosis, muscle tends to get most of the ketone bodies for fuel, but as things proceed, more ketone bodies are diverted to the brain. The ketone bodies can reduce the need for glucose by more than half.

A low-carbohydrate diet will supply the protein for glucose synthesis, but the adaptive mechanisms that have evolved to spare protein in starvation will remain operative—so the state of the body with reduced carbohydrate intake is not unlike that in starvation. This is why George Cahill, who did the pioneering work in ketone bodies and starvation, described the Atkins diet as a "high-calorie starvation diet."

There is no requirement for dietary glucose, but what is the requirement for glucose in the body as a fuel? The number that you see in the literature is 130 grams per day, and it's a number with a strange history. In George Cahill's classic study on the response to starvation,[3] it was found that this was the amount of glucose consumed by the brain under normal conditions—that is, before the starvation phase of the experiment began. After several days of starvation, however, the amount was found to be substantially less, in the range of 50 grams per day (at this point, the glucose was obviously not coming from diet, since it was measured under starvation conditions). Somehow, nutritionists picked up on the baseline 130 grams per day figure and even morphed this into a dietary requirement. Cahill told my colleague Eugene Fine that by the time he realized this had happened it was too late to stop it. The mistake has since spread throughout the literature, compounded by the suggestion that not only do you need 130 grams of glucose (not always true), but that you need to get that 130 grams specifically from diet (never true).

In summary, the brain and CNS require about 50 grams per day of glucose, and under conditions of low glucose, other fuels—namely, ketone bodies—might become more important. Many questions remain unanswered, however. Who is directing all this? How does the fat cell know when to provide fatty acids to the liver? How does the liver know when to make ketone bodies, and how many? What controls whether glucose is burned for energy or stored as fat? And thus we see the real problem in the study of metabolism. A metabolic map, like any map, only tells you about possible routes; it doesn't tell you where the traffic lights are, and it might or might not tell you where the traffic cops are. What we do know is that the most important of the traffic regulators, not surprisingly at this point, is insulin.

The Role of Insulin

Insulin is an anabolic, or building up, hormone. Of the numerous regulators of metabolism, insulin is the most important, targeting a number of organs and processes. One of its primary effects is blocking the breakdown of fat to fatty acids. Indirectly, insulin inhibits breakdown of fat and favors fat storage, as well as glucose storage in the form of glycogen. Uptake into muscle is also stimulated by recruitment of the glucose transporters, the GLUT4 receptors. GLUT4 is described as an "insulin-dependent receptor," and clearance through this receptor was once considered to be the main effect of glucose, though it is now thought to be secondary. Overall, insulin clears glucose and stores it, catalyzes fat storage, and builds new proteins. Physiologically, it is a sign of good times.

Looking ahead, in the case of diabetes, where there may be an absence of insulin (type 1) or poor response to circulating insulin (type 2), the effects on lipid metabolism might be more important than the effects on carbohydrate metabolism, even though the primary problem rests with inadequate response to ingested glucose (contained in sugar or starch). The most immediate and salient feature of diabetes, however, is the hyperglycemia (high blood glucose) due to a failure to prevent hepatic production from the breakdown of glycogen and the synthesis of new glucose via gluconeogenesis. The addition of dietary glucose on top of this will obviously make things worse.

Ketone Bodies, Ketoacidosis, and Insulin

Ketone bodies are acids, and as such, circulation must be protected against acidosis in their presence. Ketosis can become very high in type 1 diabetes, and ketoacidosis is one of the major threats of untreated type 1. So how is ketoacidosis prevented in people without diabetes and why does it occur in those with the disease? The idea is that, like most processes in metabolism, ketone-body synthesis and utilization is controlled by feedback loops. Here's the process:

1. When glucose is low, insulin is low and glucagon is high (in cases of starvation or low-carbohydrate diet). This leads to disinhibition of lipolysis in the fat cells, the process of fat breakdown that is normally repressed by insulin. The net effect is that fatty acid is increased and exported in the blood. Fatty acids in the blood, again, are referred to as free fatty acids (FFA) or nonesterified fatty acids (NEFA).
2. The fatty acids are oxidized in the liver. Fatty acids are degraded by β-oxidation, which chops off two-carbon acetyl-CoA molecules stepwise.
3. Acetyl-CoA is the substrate for energy metabolism in liver and other cells, but . . .

4. As acetyl-CoA increases, it is converted to the four-carbon ketone bodies β-hydroxybutyrate and acetoacetate, and is transported to other tissues where it regenerates acetyl-CoA. As before, ketone bodies are a way of transporting acetyl-CoA.

5. Ketone bodies regulate their own production in several ways. One way is to reduce the FFA that goes to the liver.

6. There are two major feedback inhibitors: Back at the adipocyte (fat cell), the level of ketonemia (ketone bodies in the blood) is sensed by receptors. When the concentration is high, the ketone bodies turn off their own synthesis—that is, they inhibit lipolysis. In addition to this direct effect, ketone bodies also stimulate secretion of insulin from the pancreas. This, in turn, inhibits lipolysis. So you're left with lower fatty acids, lower acetyl-CoA in the liver, and lower ketone bodies.

7. If glucose is still low, lipolysis is increased, and fatty acids "go back up."

8. Which process happens first? Well, it all happens at once. The whole system might not move because it is locked into the steady state of interlocking effects of glucose, insulin, ketone bodies, fatty acids, and everything else. The level of insulin biases the whole system in one direction or the other, but everything controls the final state.

A person with type 1 diabetes, lacking insulin, cannot exert feedback control and is therefore in danger of ketoacidosis—since the ketone bodies are acids, high levels will increase acidity.

An electronic amplifier provides a good analogy. The input from your sound system can be amplified greatly, in which case the amplifier is said to have very-high open-loop gain. Such a large signal, however, will also amplify the distortion: Small changes will cause large noise in the output. The distortion is dealt with by feeding some of the output back into the amplifier in the opposite direction of the incoming signal—so-called negative feedback. The gain (amplification) is thus greatly reduced, but the fidelity is increased. The process is similar in metabolism, where you don't want big fluctuations. In type 1 diabetes, however, the fatty-acid signal cannot be adequately controlled. It's analogous to hooking your system up to an electric guitar whose signal can't be controlled and is said to drive your amplifier into saturation. You are left with an increase in distortion.

CHAPTER 6

Sugar, Fructose, and Fructophobia

Whatever your degree of interest in nutrition, you are likely familiar with the media's crusade against sugar. There are now numerous scientific articles, picked up by the popular media, with titles like "Consuming Fructose-Sweetened, Not Glucose-Sweetened, Beverages Increases Visceral Adiposity and Lipids and Decreases Insulin Sensitivity in Overweight/Obese Humans."[1] The sudden and pervasive spread of high-fructose corn syrup (HFCS) has made fructose a particular object of fear and loathing, despite the fact that HFCS has about the same proportions of fructose and glucose (55:45) as table sugar (50:50). The strange bedfellows in this political movement include Michael Bloomberg, the former mayor of New York, and Robert Lustig, a pediatric endocrinologist. Exaggeration and alternative facts are the standard: Bloomberg claimed that banning large bottles of soda would solve the problem of obesity, and Lustig told us that sugar was as bad as alcohol or cocaine. How do we make sense of all this?

We have always known that if you sit around all day eating candy, you will get fat. Conversely, cutting down on sugar, which is a carbohydrate, will contribute to weight loss and other benefits of a low-carbohydrate diet. The extent to which sugar, that is, sucrose, or its component fructose (sucrose is half glucose and half fructose), has a unique role in obesity and other effects of carbohydrate is not well understood. However the observed differences are not large, and as discussed below, on a low-carbohydrate diet, any fructose that is ingested will be converted to glucose.

The problem with the numerous scientific papers claiming that fructose is dangerous is that they are all carried out against a background of 55 percent total carbohydrate diets. If you are going to remove carbohydrates from your diet, you might want to know whether fructose or glucose should be eliminated—that is, whether sugar is better, worse, or the same as starch. What these studies show you, instead, is how bad it is to add fructose on top of existing nutrients, or to replace glucose with fructose. It is not reasonable to think that we will solve things by keeping a high-carbohydrate diet and switching from orange juice to the whole-grain bread that always seems slightly indigestible (at least to some of us).

The problem is that we don't really have an answer when it comes to fructose. For people with diabetes or metabolic syndrome, or even those who are overweight, the data are clear: Total carbohydrate restriction—any carbohydrate—is the most effective therapy. Yet we don't know the extent to which removing fructose is a player in these therapeutic effects—because of the insulin effect, if you have diabetes, it is almost always better to remove starch than to remove sugar. The sugars are interconvertible and effects differ depending on conditions. You don't need credentials to do science, but what professionals do know is that you can't simply make guesses. Because of the complexities—depending on conditions more than half of ingested fructose is turned to glucose—you can't extrapolate from isolated experiments. Sometimes, you need the data. Biochemists are rare in nutrition because we simply don't know enough. I continue to admit that I am just about the only biochemist dumb enough to get involved here.

In Defense of Sugar (and Fructose)

Writing a "defense" of sugar seems very odd. In some ways, it's in the same vein as the defenses of saturated fat that I have written in the past. In those cases, I stressed the need for perspective. People have been making and eating cheese for as long as they knew how. What am I defending? Eggs Benedict? Béarnaise sauce? Soppressata sausage? These have been part of our culture for generations. Were we really supposed to believe that some recent earth-shattering scientific discovery meant we'd been consuming poison all along? It didn't seem to make sense, and in fact, the science was very poor, sometimes embarrassingly poor. It's the same case with fructose. Sugar is a food, and while nobody denies that many in the population are plagued by overconsumption due to excessive availability, it is still a feature of la cuisine, haute and otherwise. Chocolate mousse is as much a part of our culture as Wagner. Some of us have to limit mousse to very small doses, but for many, that is also true of Wagner.

The Threat of Fructophobia

Rob Lustig is a nice guy. Everybody says this before criticizing his increasingly unrestrained crusade against sugar. He is almost as ubiquitous as HFCS itself. His YouTube and *60 Minutes* performances, among others, have raised him to the standard of scientific spokesperson against fructose. One of Lustig's YouTube videos begins with the question, "What do the Atkins diet and Japanese food have in common?" The answer is supposed to be the absence of sugar but, of course, that isn't true.

Sugar is an easy target. These days, if you say "sugar," people think of oft-vilified foods such as Pop-Tarts or Twinkies, rather than red wine poached pears or tamagoyaki, the sweet omelet that is a staple in Bento Boxes. Here's a question, though: If you look on the ingredients list for Pop-Tarts, what is the first ingredient, the one in largest amount? It's not sugar; it's enriched flour. When I posted this on my blog, one person claimed that although flour is the first ingredient, if you add up the high-fructose corn syrup, dextrose, and other types of sugar, their sum is larger. Some have indeed suggested that this is a strategy to hide total sugar content. It's an interesting idea, but easily disproven: The label clearly says that there are 38 grams of total carbohydrate and only 17 grams of sugar.

Whether or not they think that carbohydrates are inherently fattening, most people agree that by focusing on fat, the nutritional establishment gave people license to overconsume carbohydrates, thus contributing to the obesity epidemic. Now, by focusing specifically on fructose, the AHA, USDA, and other organizations are giving implicit license to overconsume starch—it's almost guaranteed since these agencies are still down on fat and protein. The additional threat is that in an environment of fructophobia, the only studies on fructose that will be funded are those with subjects consuming high levels of carbohydrate. In such studies the two sugars, glucose and fructose, interact metabolically and sometimes synergistically, so deleterious effects of fructose are likely to be found. The results will likely be generalized to all conditions, and as with lipophobia, there will be no null hypothesis.

The barrier to introducing some common sense into the discussion is, again, that we really don't have the answers. We don't have enough data. The idea that fructose is a unique agent in increasing triglycerides (fat in the blood) is greatly exaggerated. High-carbohydrate diets lead to high triglycerides, and there are indeed conditions where sugar has a worse effect than starch, but the differences between the effects of fructose specifically and those of carbohydrates in general are small. The greatest threat of fructophobia is that we won't find out what the real effect of fructose is. Furthermore, the two regimes being compared in current studies are both high in carbohydrate, and because the absolute level of the triglycerides is high in both cases, it is likely that the biggest difference would be seen if either of the outcomes were compared to the results of a low-carbohydrate diet.

The single most important question to ask with regard to sugar is this: For a person on the so-called standard, high-carbohydrate American diet, is it better to replace carbohydrate (any carbohydrate) with fat (any fat except trans-fat), or to replace fructose with glucose? Ignoring subtleties, to a first approximation, which is better?

We might not know the answer to that question in every case, but the studies that have been done clearly indicate that replacing carbohydrate with fat is more beneficial. We also know that ethanol is not processed like fructose despite what many claim on the internet. Although the pathways converge, like almost all substrates that are used for energy at the entry to the TCA cycle, they are different. It's just not true that there is a similarity. We also know that although some claim glycogen is not formed from fructose, and Lustig shows a metabolic pathway from which glycogen is absent, fructose does actually give rise to glycogen. Under most conditions, fructose is a preferred substrate for glycogen synthesis. (In fact, for some period in the history of chemistry, fructose was primarily considered a "glycogenic substrate.") Of course, fructose must first be converted to glucose. Claude Bernard knew that fructose could give rise to glycogen, but he couldn't understand why he wasn't able to find any fructose within the glycogen itself.

To return to the comparison that is often made between sugar and ethanol, it is possible that sugar and ethanol have behavioral effects in common, but this is not due to similarities in metabolism. Moreover, the behavioral effects are not even settled within the psychology community:

Alcoholism is far different from sugar addiction, if there is such a thing. While there is no definite agreement, *addictive* has formal definitions in behavioral psychology, and polishing off the whole bag of chocolate chip cookies might not technically qualify as addictive behavior. Some restraint is necessary. Alcohol-associated liver disease is a well-characterized, life-threatening condition, and many people do die from it. The idea that fructose can have the same effect, either physically or psychologically, has no basis in science and is deeply offensive to people who have had personal experience with alcohol-related illness and death.

In the end, nobody has ever been admitted to a hospital for an overdose of fructose. People might say that your diabetes was caused by fructose consumption, but you can't be admitted to a hospital on somebody's opinion of what you did wrong. There is no diagnosis called "fructose poisoning." If you are admitted to the hospital for type 2 diabetes, that is the diagnosis.

The Threat of Policy

The numerous scientific papers that find something wrong with fructose may have had little impact on people's behavior, but possibly for that reason, the fructophobes have taken new steps. Convinced of the correctness of their position, they have taken their case to politicians who are always eager to tax and regulate. There is an obvious sense of déjà vu as another group of experts tries to use the American population as guinea pigs for a massive population experiment, along the lines of the low-fat fiasco under which we still suffer (not to mention the historical example of alcohol prohibition). It is not just that the lipophobe movement had unintended consequences (think margarine and trans-fats) but rather that, as numerous people have pointed out, the science was never there for low-fat to begin with. In other words, before science is turned into policy, we have to address the question of whether the science is any good to begin with.

Fructose in Perspective

Contrary to popular myth, the "Twinkie Defense" of Harvey Milk's murderer Dan White did not argue that the defendant was possessed by some kind of sugar rush. Rather, the defense claimed that he was propelled to homicide by his depressed state, and that this deranged mental condition was indicated by his consumption of junk food. (He had previously been a health nut.) It was a strange defense, because most of us think of depressives as going for suicide rather than homicide—but in any case, sugar did not make him do it.

Fructose is a normal nutrient and metabolite. It is a carbohydrate and it is metabolized in the metabolic pathways of carbohydrate processing. If nothing else, your body makes a certain amount of fructose. Fructose, not music (the food of love according to Shakespeare), is the preferred fuel of sperm cells. Fructose formed in the eye can be a risk but its cause is generally very high glucose. The polyol reaction involves sequential conversion of glucose to sorbitol and then to fructose.

One truly bizarre twist in the campaign against fructose was the study by Miguel Lanaspa and his colleagues[2] that attempted to show that the deleterious effects of glucose were due to its conversion to fructose via the polyol reaction. The paper was technical, but many people reading it in *Nature* don't think that the conclusion really followed from the data—it would be a major change in metabolic thinking, and if it were true, it would have been accepted. If the idea has not actually been excluded, then it must be some expression of the need to say that, somehow or another, everything bad is caused by fructose.

My review with Eugene Fine, "Fructose in Perspective," was published in 2013 in *Nutrition and Metabolism* with the following conclusion:

> We all agree that reducing sugar intake as a way of reducing calories or limiting carbohydrates, is a good thing, especially for children, but it is important to remember that fructose and sucrose are carbohydrates. We know well the benefits of reducing total carbohydrate. How much of such benefits can be attributed to removing sugar is unknown. The major point is that these sugars are rapidly incorporated into normal carbohydrate metabolism. In some sense, any unique effects of sucrose that are observed are due to fructose acting as a kind of super-glucose.[3]

Again, the threat is thinking that fructose is sufficiently different from glucose that substituting glucose for fructose is guaranteed to be better. It's

The Evolutionary Argument

It is still frequently said that our metabolism is not designed to handle the high input of fructose that was absent in our evolution and that is present in our current environment. Although fructose might not have been widely available in Paleolithic times, that doesn't mean that high consumption was uncommon. It is likely that, for our ancestors, finding the rare berry bush was like finding a coupon for Häagen-Dazs. Moderation was not the key word. While few would argue that wide availability or high consumption is without risk, it is important to hew to the science. There is a big difference between saying that continued ingestion of high sugar (or high carbohydrates, or high anything) is not good, and saying that we do not have the metabolic machinery to deal with high intake, or that it is a foreign, toxic substance.

not. Our review was a technical analysis of the literature, summarized in a rather complicated figure showing what is known of the two sugars. That figure might not be easily accessible to everybody, but figure 6.1, a simplified version of the one in the study, explains some of the key points. Fructose and glucose follow separate paths initially, but both six-carbon sugars are broken down to three-carbon fragments, the triose phosphates. These triose phosphates are the intermediates in the effects of high carbohydrate ingestion: high plasma triglycerides and low HDL ("good cholesterol").

The question for anybody who wants to attribute special properties to fructose is how an atom in a triose phosphate knows whether it came from fructose or from glucose. Of course, it doesn't, and the outstanding feature of fructose metabolism is that it is part of glucose metabolism. Figure 6.1 shows the path by which fructose can be turned into glucose, and under the appropriate conditions, into glycogen. As much as 60 percent of ingested fructose can be converted to glucose via gluconeogenesis. So, is there

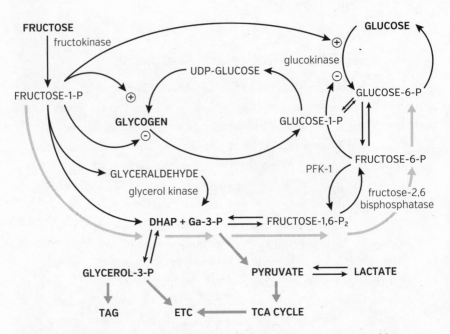

Figure 6.1. A model of hepatic fructose metabolism. Key notes include: (1) Fructose stimulates glycogen storage; (2) fructose and glucose share common intermediates; (3) fructose can be converted to glucose; (4) ingested fructose calls for more glucose; and (5) generally, the liver expects glucose and fructose to come in together.

really no difference between fructose and glucose? It turns out that the differences are small, and those that exist are due to kinetic (rate) effects rather than overall pattern of processing. Fructose is rapidly processed. Technically, fructokinase, the first enzyme to process fructose, has a low Km, which refers to the fact that it doesn't take much fructose to get its metabolism going at a high rate. The carbons from fructose appear in the triose phosphates very quickly. So, if one wanted to make a grand statement, it might be that fructose is, as we called it, a kind of super-glucose.

This is not an academic conclusion, however. We still need to know whether sugar acts primarily as a carbohydrate. Again, if we remove sugar and replace it with starch, how will the results compare with the many trials that show benefits of removing carbohydrate across the board and replacing it with fat? Nobody has directly made the comparison. The experiment has never been done. Experiments with real low-carbohydrate diets give far more dramatic results than those that replace fructose with glucose.

One important phenomenon to note: The amount of glucose in the human diet is always greater than the amount of fructose (see figure 6.2). It is unlikely that anybody eats only sugar and no starch (which, again, is all glucose), and even HFCS has only slightly more fructose than glucose. Pure glucose is used for various effects in commercial food preparation. You will therefore almost never see pure fructose in the absence of glucose in the human diet. Moreover, ingested fructose triggers an increase in the glucokinase, the first glucose-processing enzyme in the liver, leading to further uptake of glucose. In other words, fructose calls for glucose—the liver expects the two sugars together. This is important, in that administering fructose alone is clearly detrimental. When it was discovered that fructose does not stimulate insulin secretion, some thought that fructose might be a good replacement for glucose for people with diabetes—again reflecting the idea that everybody needs sugar to be happy. It turned out that consuming fructose without glucose is dangerous. It is important to recognize, however, that the effects of fructose alone are not comparable to those of fructose in combination with glucose.

In demonizing fructose across the board, we have to ask whether we are making the same rush to judgment that we did with fat. We said that dietary fat would give you heart disease, and a cascade of changes in medical practice flowed from that, but it has never been shown that fat gives you heart disease. A whole human population went all out to replace fat with carbohydrate, and this led to an increase in obesity and diabetes. Carbohydrate restriction remains the best strategy for obesity, diabetes, and metabolic syndrome. The specific contribution of removal of fructose or sucrose to this effect remains unknown. *Unknown* is the key word.

Sweetener Consumption

What about sweetener consumption? Surprisingly, it hasn't gone up as much as you might have thought—about 15 percent, according to the USDA. One question is whether this increase is disproportionately due to fructose. The data show that, in fact, the ratio of fructose to glucose has remained constant over the last forty years. While sugar or HFCS is the main sweetener, pure glucose is sometimes used in the food industry and has remained at a constant 20 percent, explaining the deviation from

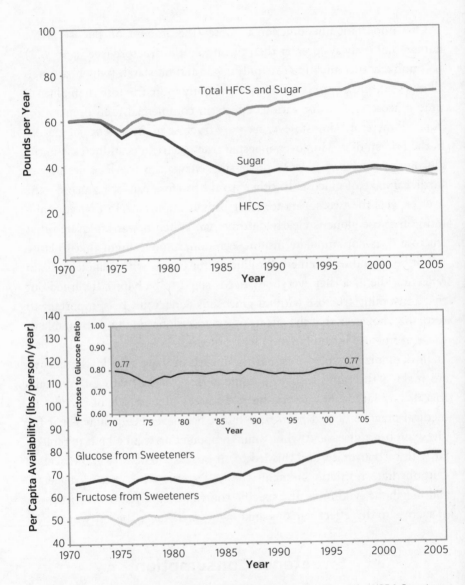

Figure 6.2. Sweetener consumption data, 1970–2005. Data from the USDA Sweetener Yearbook tables and the USDA Food Availability Data System.

1:1, which would be expected (see figure 6.2). There is, however, more glucose than fructose in the food supply. One might argue that despite the constant ratio, the absolute increase in fructose has a more pernicious effect than the increased glucose—but, of course, you would have to prove that. Figures 6.1 and 6.2 suggest that you would have to be careful in determining whether the effect of increased sweetener is due to fructose or to glucose, or whether it is the effect of one on the other, or the effect of insulin and other hormones on both.

Scapegoats

For a good example of the hyperbole surrounding discussion of fructose, consider an article in *Mother Jones* by Gary Taubes and Cristin Kearns Couzens called "Big Sugar's Sweet Little Lies."[4] The article is a fascinating, well-researched story of how the sugar industry has pushed its products, but the connection the authors make to the tobacco industry's attempts to bury information and maintain profits is an overreach. I suspect one does not have to look hard for industries that try to sell their product by underhanded means, but the ethical problems in the case of tobacco were related to the product, not its promotion. Sugar does not functionally resemble tobacco in any way. The goal, of course, is to tax or otherwise impose punishment for sugar consumption—the first reaction of politicians is to punish and tax. The decline in cigarette smoking is cited as the effect of taxation. The question of whether reduction in cigarette consumption was a response to financial pressure or education is testable, however: If the former case is true, reduction in smoking should be greater in lower-income economic groups, and it should be opposite in the latter case (sources such as the Gallup polls show the latter case is true). The *Mother Jones's* piece described a large rise in consumption of sugar sweeteners that was accompanied, in turn, by "a surge in the chronic diseases increasingly linked to sugar." You can't really expect a popular article to stand up to academic analysis, but the sentence is tricky—really illogical. It says that "the increase" in sugar is linked to diseases "linked to sugar." You can't use "linked" twice. The link of chronic disease to sugar is exactly what's in question. The graphics in the article tried to bring out the statistics, but the presentation is misleading. *Mother Jones* is not *Annalen der Physik*, of course, but some degree of precision is still required. In fact, the increase in the past thirty years is quite small. Using the numbers in the article:

$$\% \text{ Increase in sugar} = 12 / 120 = 10\%$$

Other data show that the increase was 15 percent, so we can even go with that number. For comparison, in a comparable time period, the increase in the United States for total carbohydrate was 23.4 percent for men and 38.4 percent for women. The idea, however, is that sugar has a very powerful, almost catalytic effect—in other words, a little increase in sugar is supposed to bring about big changes in health. So what happened in the thirty years that is presumed to have been a consequence of the 9 percent increase in added sugars? Again, from the figure in the paper:

% Increase in diabetes   =   4.3 / 2.5 =   172%
% Increase US children who are obese = 11.4 / 5.5 = 207.2%
% Increase US adults who are obese   = 20.7 /   15 =   138%

Is fructose that powerful? If it is, the recommended reduction would certainly be a good thing, but how likely is it that fructose was truly the root of these increases, and if it is that powerful, could it ever be adequately reduced? A 9 percent or even 15 percent increase in sugar consumption is supposed to have caused a major increase in obesity and diabetes; the absolute changes are small, but still significant since these statistics represent the entire population. The experiment to test whether fructose is actually that powerful would be easy to conduct: Compare removal of fructose with removal of glucose and the results should be evident. Again, that experiment hasn't been done. Why not? We have good experiments showing that if you take out carbohydrates and put in fat, you get significant benefit. If fructose is the most harmful of the carbohydrates, it should not be hard to show that it was fructose that was the controlling player in these comparisons. It is surprising, and perhaps even suspicious, that the experiment hasn't been done.

CHAPTER 7

Saturated Fat

On Your Plate or in Your Blood?

A high-fat diet in the presence of carbohydrate is different than a high-fat diet in the presence of low-carbohydrate. Failure to understand this principle, and the resulting failure to adequately test the effect exerted by carbohydrate, stands as a major source of confusion. Numerous reports in the medical and popular literature describe the effect of a "high-fat diet" or even "a single high-fat meal." The source of the high fat, however, might be a slice of carrot cake, a Big Mac, or something else that is also very high in carbohydrate.

On the subject of saturated fat, the studies from Jeff Volek's laboratory, then at the University of Connecticut, provide the most telling evidence. Science does not run on majority rule. The total number of experiments is less important than the scientific design of the individual trials and whether it is easy to interpret their results. A study from Volek's lab on forty volunteers with metabolic syndrome provides a classic case, carefully controlled and unambiguous.

Particularly striking, the study found that when the blood of volunteers was assayed for saturated fatty acids, those who had been on a low-carbohydrate diet had lower levels than those on an isocaloric low-fat diet—this despite the fact that the low-carbohydrate diet had three times the amount of dietary saturated fat as the low-fat diet. How was this possible? Well, that's what metabolism does. For those on the low-carbohydrate diet, the saturated fat was oxidized, while the low-fat group was making new saturated fatty acid. Volek's former student, Cassandra Forsythe, extended the idea by showing how, even under eucaloric conditions (no weight loss), dietary fat has relatively little impact on fat in the blood.[1]

A barrier to understanding the role of saturated fat rests with the emphasis on "diets," where it is impossible to come to an agreement on definitions and where an accidental or individual response might happen to work for an individual or small group of people (e.g., the generic ad hoc grapefruit diet). We would do better by speaking, instead, of basic principles. The key principle is that dietary carbohydrate, directly or indirectly, through insulin and other hormones, controls what happens to ingested and stored fatty acids. Carbohydrate has a catalytic effect—it controls what happens to other nutrients. The fat in the Big Mac will not constitute any risk if you chuck the bun. You are not what you eat. You are what you do with what you eat.

The question of saturated fat is critical. The scientific evidence shows that dietary saturated fat, in general, has no effect on cardiovascular disease, obesity, or probably anything else—but plasma saturated fatty acids do. In particular, plasma saturated fatty acids can provide a cellular signal, and they exacerbate insulin resistance. If you study dietary saturated fatty acids under conditions where carbohydrate is high, or, more importantly, if your study effects are in rodents, where plasma fat better correlates with dietary fat, then you will confuse plasma fat with dietary fat. There is a real difference.

To understand the problem, recall that strictly speaking, there are only saturated fatty acids (SFAs). What is called "saturated fat" simply means those fats that have a high percentage of SFAs. Things that we identify as "saturated fats," such as butter, usually contain only 50 percent saturated fatty acids. Coconut oil is probably the only fat that is almost entirely saturated fatty acids, but because those acids are medium-chain length, they are usually considered a special case.

In Volek's experiment, forty overweight subjects were randomly assigned to one of two diets[2]: a very low-carbohydrate ketogenic diet (VLCKD), which provided a macronutrient distribution of about 12 percent carbohydrate, 59 percent fat, and 28 percent protein; or a low-fat diet (LFD) composed of 56 percent carbohydrate, 24 percent fat, and 20 percent protein. The group was unusual in that they were all overweight and would all be characterized as having metabolic syndrome. All subjects demonstrated the features of atherogenic dyslipidemia, a subset of metabolic syndrome markers that describes a poor lipid profile: high triacylglycerol (TAG), low HDL-C, and high small-dense LDL (so-called pattern B).

What's striking in Volek's work is the difference in weight loss between the two diet regimens. Participants in the study were not specifically counseled to reduce calories but both groups spontaneously reduced caloric intake. (Apparently, people in diet studies tend to automatically reduce calories.) However the level of weight loss between the two groups, due to the macronutrient composition of the plans, was dramatically different. People on the VLCKD lost twice as much weight on average as those on the LFD despite the similar caloric intake. Although there was substantial individual variation (see figure 9.2 on page 134), nine of twenty subjects in the VLCKD group lost 10 percent of their starting body weight, more weight than was lost by any of the subjects in the LFD group. In fact, nobody following the LFD lost as much weight as the average for the low-carbohydrate group. The major differences between the VLCKD and LFD groups appeared in the changes in whole body fat mass: 5.7 kilograms and 3.7 kilograms, respectively.

It is generally believed that deposition of fat in the abdominal region is more undesirable than subcutaneous fat. Abdominal fat was found to be reduced more in subjects on the VLCKD than in subjects following the LFD (-828 grams versus -506 grams). Volek's study thus provides one of the more dramatic demonstrations of the benefits of carbohydrate restriction for weight loss. Similar results had preceded it, though. Those preceding studies had frequently been disparaged for increasing the amount of saturated fat as a sort of automatic criticism (whether or not any particular study actually increased saturated fat). Although the original "concern" was increased plasma cholesterol, eventually saturated fat became a generalized villain, and insofar as the science was concerned, the effects of plasma saturated fat were assumed to be due to dietary saturated fat. The surprising outcome of Volek's study was that there was, in fact, inverse correlation between dietary and plasma SFA. It was surprising because the effect was so clear-cut that no statistics were needed, and because an underlying mechanism could explain the results.

On Your Plate or in Your Blood?

In Volek's study the dietary intake of saturated fat for the people on the VLCKD averaged out to 36 grams per day, threefold higher than that of the people on the LFD (12 grams per day). When the relative proportions of circulating SFAs in the triglyceride and cholesterol ester fractions were determined, however, they were actually lower in the low-carbohydrate group. Seventeen of twenty subjects on the VLCKD showed a decrease in total saturates, while the other three already had low values at baseline. In distinction, only half of the subjects consuming the LFD showed a decrease in SFA. When the absolute fasting TAG levels are taken into account (low-carbohydrate diets reliably reduce TAG), the absolute concentration of total saturates in plasma TAG was reduced by 57 percent in the low-carbohydrate group compared to only 24 percent reduction in the low-fat group—again, this is despite the fact that LFD group had reduced their dietary saturated fat intake. How could this happen? The low-fat group reduced their SFA intake by one-third, yet had more SFA in their blood than the low-carbohydrate group who had actually increased intake. Metabolism is about change. Chemistry is about transformation.

De Novo Lipogenesis

To review the major features of metabolism bearing on fat, there are roughly two kinds of fuel: glucose and acetyl-CoA. The big principle is that you can make acetyl-CoA from glucose, but in most cases you can't make glucose from acetyl-CoA—or, more generally, you can make fat from glucose but you can't make glucose from fat. So, how do you make fat from glucose? Part of the picture is the process of making new fatty acids, known as de novo lipogenesis (DNL), or more accurately de novo fatty acid synthesis. The mechanism for making new fatty acids is, in a rough sort of way, the reverse of breaking them down. You successively patch together two-carbon acetyl-CoA units until you reach the chain length of sixteen carbons: palmitic acid, the saturated fatty acid that was found in higher concentrations in the subjects on low-fat diets in Volek's experiment. Palmitic acid can then be elongated to stearic acid (18:0) or desaturated to the unsaturated fatty acid, palmitoleic acid (16:1-n7, 16 carbons, one unsaturation at carbon 7).

The critical part is getting the process going. The first step is the formation of a three-carbon compound called malonyl-CoA, a process under the control of insulin. Malonyl-CoA enters into the synthetic process and simultaneously prevents transport of fatty acid into the mitochondrion where it would be oxidized. If you are making new fatty acid, you don't want to burn it. New fatty acid is a reasonable explanation for the increased SFA in the low-fat group. The low-carbohydrate group, on the other hand, would be expected to have higher insulin levels on average, encouraging diversion of calories into fatty acid synthesis and repressing oxidation. How could this be tested?

It turns out that the unsaturated fatty acid, palmitoleic acid (16:1-n7), is not common in the diet and therefore stands as a good indicator of synthesis. The same enzyme that catalyzes conversion of palmitic acid also catalyzes conversion of stearic acid (18:0) to the unsaturated fatty acid oleic acid (18:1n-7), as in olive oil. The enzyme in question is named for the second reaction, stearoyl-CoA desaturase-1 (SCD-1). SCD-1 is membrane-bound, which means that it is not swimming around the cell looking for fatty acids, but instead is closely tied to DNL (waiting at the end of the assembly line so to speak), and preferentially desaturates newly formed fatty acids: palmitic acid to palmitoleic acid and stearic to oleic. It is unsurprising, then, that the data from Volek's experiment show a 31 percent decrease in palmitoleic acid (16:1n-7) in the blood of subjects on the low-carbohydrate group with little overall change in the average response in the low-fat group. The low-fat group was making saturated fatty acid more than the low-carbohydrate group.

Saturated Fat in Your Blood

Cassandra Forsythe, Volek's student at the time, extended this work to an experiment on weight maintenance. It is commonly claimed that the physiologic effects of low-carbohydrate diets are linked to weight loss rather than to an inherent response to reduction in carbohydrate, so it is important to tackle this objection. In her experiment, men were assigned to one of two different weight-maintaining diets, both low in carbohydrate, for six weeks. The first of the diets was designed to be high in SFA (dairy fat and eggs), and the other was designed to be higher in unsaturated fat from both polyunsaturated (PUFA) and monounsaturated (MUFA) fatty acids (fish, nuts, omega-3 enriched eggs, and olive oil). For the SFA-carbohydrate-restricted diet, the relative percentages of SFA, MUFA, and PUFA were 31, 21, and 5, respectively. For the UFA diet, the percentages were 17, 25, and 15. The results as stated in Forsythe's study:

The most striking finding was the lack of association between dietary SFA intake and plasma SFA concentrations. Compared to baseline, a *doubling* of saturated fat intake on the CRD-SFA (carbohydrate-restricted diet with high saturated fatty acid) did not increase plasma SFA in any of the lipid fractions, and when saturated fat was only moderately increased on the CRD-UFA, the proportion of SFA in plasma TAG was reduced from 31.06% to 27.48 mol%. Since plasma TAG was also reduced, the total SFA concentration in plasma TAG was decreased by 47% after the CRD-UFA, similar to the 57% decrease we observed in overweight men and women after 12 week of a hypocaloric CRD.[3]

The bottom line: Dietary carbohydrate, rather than dietary SFA, controls plasma SFA. Therefore, while it is widely held that the type of fat is more important than the amount, this is not a universal principle, and it becomes less important if carbohydrates are low. But what about the amount? A widely cited paper by Raatz et al.[4] suggested, as indicated by the title, that "Total Fat Intake Modifies Plasma Fatty Acid Composition in Humans." The data in the paper, however, show that the differences between high-fat and low-fat were, in fact, minimal. How can you say one thing when your data show something else? One doesn't know what was on the authors' minds, and maybe they interpreted things differently, but in general it seems that the literature takes an approach similar to that of lawyers: If the jury buys it, it doesn't matter whether or not it's true. In scientific publishing, the jurors are the reviewers and the editors. If they are already convinced of the conclusion, if there is no voir dire, you will surely win the case.

The bottom line is that distribution of types of fatty acid in plasma is more dependent on the level of dietary carbohydrate consumption than the level or type of dietary fat consumption. The work of Volek and Forsythe provides a good reason to focus on the carbohydrate content of your diet. What about the type of carbohydrate, though? In other words, is glycemic index important? Is fructose as bad as they say? Consistent with the small perturbation caused by fructose compared to glucose, as shown in the previous chapter, we have a good general principle: No change in the type of macronutrient—carbohydrate or fat—will ever have the same kind of effect as replacing carbohydrate across the board with fat.

CHAPTER 8

Hunger

What It Is, What to Do About It

The reporter from *Men's Health* asked me: "You finish dinner, even a satisfying low-carb dinner"—he is a low-carbohydrate person himself—"you are sure you ate enough but you are still hungry. What do you do?" I gave him good advice: "Think of a perfectly broiled steak or steamed lobster with butter—some high protein, relatively high-fat meal that you usually like. If that doesn't sound good, you are not hungry. You might want to keep eating. You might want something sweet. You might want to feel something rolling around in your mouth, but you are not hungry. Find something else to do—push-ups are good. If the steak does sound good, you might want to eat. Practically speaking, you might want to keep hard boiled eggs, kielbasa, something filling, around (and, of course, you don't want cookies in the house)." I think this was good practical advice. My recommendation was based on the satiating effects of protein food sources, or perhaps the nonsatiating, or binge-inducing effect of carbohydrate. All this raises a larger question, though: What is hunger?

We grow up thinking that hunger is our body's way of telling us that we need food, but for most of us that is not the case. Few of us are so fit, or have so little body fat, or are so active, that our bodies start calling for energy if we miss lunch. Conversely, those of us who really like food generally hold to the philosophy that "any fool can eat when they're hungry." Passing up a really good chocolate mousse just because you are not hungry is like . . . well, I don't know what it's like. Of course, if you are on a low-carbohydrate diet, you might pass it up for dietary reasons, or at least restrain yourself from eating too much.

Getting to the point here, if I presented you with a multiple-choice question that asked what hunger is, the answer would be "all of the above."

We feel hunger when we haven't eaten for a while; we feel hunger if the food looks good; we feel hunger if we are in a social situation in which eating is going on (the spread of petits fours that were in the lobby at the break in an obesity conference, the congressional prayer breakfast, or the Pavlovian lunch bell).

Or we might eat because we think it is time to eat. This point was made by the Restoration poet and rake, John Wilmot, Earl of Rochester. Wilmot is famous for his bawdy poetry, raunchy even by today's standards, but his "Satyr against Reason and Mankind," which is more commonly included in texts on eighteenth-century literature, makes fun of dumb rules and phony reason:

> My reason is my friend, yours is a cheat;
> Hunger calls out, my reason bids me eat;
> Perversely, yours your appetite does mock:
> This asks for food, that answers, "What's o'clock?"
> This plain distinction, sir, your doubt secures:
> 'Tis not true reason I despise, but yours.

Americans have not conquered this problem, and we may in fact have made it worse. A diet experiment invariably includes a snack as if it has the same standing as breakfast, lunch, and dinner (anecdotally, the number of people who prefer to go without breakfast suggests that that meal is at least not for everyone). Visitors remark on how Americans are eating all the time, not just at meals. If you maintain such a habit, it doesn't take long until you are hungry all the time.

Different people have different responses to external cues. In experiments in which subjects are interrogated, but incidentally have snacks available—a bowl of crackers on the table, for example—it is not surprising that thin people regulate their intake by the clock on the wall. Overweight people, in distinction, are less sensitive to the clock and dip into the snacks even if "it's almost dinner time." Similarly, at Union Theological Seminary in New York, the school for training rabbis, it is the overweight students who adhere better to fasting on high holy days. Consumption is less connected to internal (physiologic) cues and external (religious) reasons can have control.

The psychologist B. F. Skinner[1] described the problem in a characteristically dense way:

> "I am hungry" may be equivalent to "I have hunger pangs," and if the verbal community had some means of observing the contractions of the stomach associated with pangs, it could pin the response to these stimuli alone. It may also be equivalent to "I am eating actively." A person who observes that he is eating voraciously may say, "I really am hungry," or, in retrospect, "I was hungrier than I thought," dismissing other evidence as unreliable. "I am hungry" may also be equivalent to "It has been a long time since I have had anything to eat," although the expression is most likely to be used in describing future behavior: "If I miss my dinner, I shall be hungry."

What Skinner's saying is that whatever the actual causes of eating behavior, the behavior itself may precede the description of the "motivation to eat." In other words, we tend to identify a feeling that is associated with eating behavior as the *cause* of the behavior. "I am hungry" may also be equivalent to "I feel like eating" in the sense of "I have felt this way before when I have started to eat." The point is that "hungry" only means you are in a situation where you are used to eating. It doesn't mean that feeling hungry will make you eat, or, more importantly, that you have to eat.

Lessons from Vagotomy

The vagus nerve contains many nerve fibers that facilitate communication between the brain and other parts of the body (a nerve is a collection of nerve cells or neurons whose long extensions or axons are referred to as fibers). Cells that send signals from the brain to distant organs are called efferent. Efferent fibers in the vagus nerve regulate the digestive tract in various ways: enlargement of the stomach, for example, or secretions from the pancreas to deal with larger volumes of food (known to doctors as accommodation). Most of the fibers in the vagus nerve are sensory afferents (afferents carry information from the body to the brain) providing sensations of satiety and hunger as well as a feeling of discomfort when we are full. (Efferent is usually pronounced "EE-ferent" to distinguish from afferents.)

Vagotomy, cutting the vagus nerve, was historically practiced as a means of controlling ulcers, and is still a target, at least experimentally, for treating obesity. Dr. John Kral at the Department of Surgery at Downstate, who has performed such operations, described to me how patients complained that they had lost their appetite. He had to explain to them that you do not have to eat all the time, and that nothing bad will happen if you miss a few meals. Hunger is a signal that you are used to eating in a particular time or situation. You are not required to answer that signal.

"You Eat Because You Are Fat"

In trying to go beyond energy balance there is a tendency to think of hunger in terms of hormones, emphasizing regulation by the hypothalamus, analogous to temperature regulation. The hormones in question are referred to as either orexigenic, increasing appetite (from the Greek: the Greek equivalent of *bon appetite* is *kali orexi*), or anorexigenic, depressing appetite. While this is part of the picture, it leads to some confusion because the endocrine approach emphasizes hormonal output from the fat cell, and in some sense bypasses the question of how the fat cell got fat in the first place—that is, how it bypasses metabolism. More importantly, for animals and humans outside of a laboratory setup, behavior overrides hormones. The analogy is not entirely accurate in that animals (and humans) regulate their temperature hormonally only to a small extent. The major control of temperature is behavioral: We put on clothes and we hide in caves.

An important aspect of this problem is the need to understand the error in "a calorie is a calorie." One critique of the energy balance model runs something like this:

$$\text{dietary carbohydrate} \rightarrow \text{insulin} \rightarrow \text{(other hormones)} \rightarrow \text{increased appetite} \rightarrow \text{greater consumption}$$

In the extreme case, the explanation might boil down to: "You don't get fat because you eat; you eat because you got fat." This doesn't make much sense. It sounds like one of the seemingly profound academic aphorism that Woody Allen was so good at parodying: "All of literature is just a footnote to Faust." I understand that it implies that the hormonal secretion from adipose tissue encourages eating—but again, it does not tell you why you got fat in the first place. It mixes up metabolism with behavior and implicitly accepts the idea that calories are what count—that it is the total energy you consume that matters, rather than how that energy is processed. Although macronutrients clearly differ in satiety, regardless of your hormonal state, if there is no food, you will not increase consumption. Also, the effects of insulin are not so clear-cut. Whereas metabolically insulin is anabolic, at the level of behavior it is probably anorexigenic in most cases.

Why do we get fat? We get fat because we eat too much of the stuff that encourages excessive weight gain. We don't know what that *stuff* is, but we know that it is not fat per se. Given the unambiguous effectiveness of carbohydrate restriction in reducing excess weight, it would be surprising if carbohydrate weren't a big part of the picture. The so-called metabolic advantage (less weight gain per calorie), where it exists, is a metabolic effect. The most likely mechanism appears to be due to the effect of insulin on rates of reaction: Anabolic (storage) steps might increase accumulation before competing feedback (breakdown) can catch up. As I will explain in chapter 9, it rests on nonequilibrium thermodynamics,[2] which recognizes the importance of rates as well as energy.

What Can You Do About It?

The suggestion at the beginning of this section was to make sure you know what kind of hunger you are talking about. Behavioral psychology stresses the difference between "tastes good," and the technical term, "reinforcing," which means that the food increases the probability that you will keep eating. Anecdotally, we all have the experience of saying, "I don't know why I ate that. It wasn't very good."

However little you eat to answer feelings of hunger, it is certainly bad advice to eat if you are not hungry. Professional nutritionists, even the Atkins website, are always telling you to have a good breakfast. Why you would want to have any "good" meal if you are trying to lose weight is not easy to answer. The nutritionists claim that without breakfast, you will eat too much at the next meal, as if in the morning you can make the rational decision to eat breakfast despite no desire for food, while at noon you are suddenly under the inexorable influence of urges beyond your control. A more reasonable way to put it would be: "If you find that you eat too much at lunch when you don't eat breakfast, then . . . ," but that is not the style of traditional nutrition.

More on Behavior

The principle in behavioral psychology is that how soon a behavior is reinforced is more important than the quality of the reinforcer. It is important to reemphasize that reinforcement is not always equivalent to reward. Reinforcement simply means increasing the likelihood that a behavior will reappear, even if that behavior doesn't feel totally good. Junk food may be reinforcing in that it will make you eat more even though you realize afterward it didn't taste that good. Taste and mouth feel are so immediately reinforcing that, in all likelihood, only aversive stimulation can work well to discourage eating. There are positive ways to look at hunger. For example: Feeling hungry may mean that your diet is working, that you really are losing weight, and therefore you might stop eating before satiation. However encouraging that notion might be, it usually can't compete well with even the smell of food. You need something strongly negative.

One of the more effective regimens is a diet strategy from Dr. Allen Fay, a psychiatrist in New York. It works like this:

1. You pick an amount of weight you want to lose in the next week; you can pick zero but, of course, you can't go up.
2. You write a check for $2,000 to an organization that you don't like (Republican National Committee, in my case) and give it to Dr. Fay. (Note: This is a personal choice. This is not a political book.)
3. If, at the end of the week, you haven't hit the weight target, he mails the check.

In some cases, Dr. Fay said, you don't even need money. One patient wrote a letter, poised to be sent to a right-to-life organization, telling

Exercise

The only thing that people in nutrition agree on is the value of exercise. While it is not as important as diet for weight loss, it does positively interact with diet and has obvious benefit. One question that comes up is when to have meals in relation to exercise. Although outside my area of expertise, and likely to be an individual thing, there is some good guidance in the following old joke:

> The couple go to the doctor and don't want to have any more children but they don't want any artificial methods of birth control. The doctor recommends exercise.
>
> Husband: Before or after?
>
> Doctor: Instead of.

them what a great job they were doing. The thought that she would get on their mailing list as a supporter was sufficiently unpleasant to keep her on target.

You pick your own threat, of course—it is not a political method. Dr. Fay suggested the American Nazi Party, but I thought that they would only buy those shabby uniforms, whereas from my perspective, the Republicans would do real damage. My relation to Dr. Fay is partly professional (although he admits there are people who are beyond psychotherapy) and partly friend. For the technique to work, you must be distant enough from the person holding the check so that they will actually mail it, but close enough that you will not consider physical violence if they do.

Imagery can help, but only up to a point. A major problem situation for dieters is that they have eaten what they want and feel satisfied, but there is still food on their plate, which they pick at until they feel sick. My approach when I felt full was to imagine spiders coming out of the food. This worked for a while, but over time I noticed that I was losing my distaste of spiders. Eating has a very strong Pavlovian component. It is not nice to fool Mother Nature.

CHAPTER 9

Beyond
"A Calorie Is a Calorie"

An Introduction to Thermodynamics

Arnold Sommerfeld was one of the great physicists in the development of quantum mechanics (theory of atomic structure). He was also generally considered to be an expert on most areas of physics. His take on thermodynamics:

> The first time I studied it, I thought that I understood it except for a few minor details.
> The second time I studied it, I thought that I didn't understand it except for a few minor details.
> The third time I studied it, I knew I didn't understand it but it didn't matter because I already knew how to use it.[1]

Can you really lose more weight on one diet than another if you consume the same number of calories? The question usually comes in response to a low-carbohydrate diet, where the so-called metabolic advantage promises you that cutting out carbohydrate will lead to reduced efficiency in storing fat. Folks go crazy when you suggest it's true. Whenever a scientific paper presents data showing that such a thing really happens—that one diet, usually low-carbohydrate, is more effective than another—somebody always jumps in to say that it is impossible, and that it would violate the laws of thermodynamics. Like the cartoon characters who run over the cliff, remain suspended in thin air, and fall only when they realize that they aren't on solid ground, somehow the data are expected to go away once thermodynamics is invoked. Of course, the data can't violate the laws of thermodynamics. The real possibility is that the data are accurate and that the critic doesn't get it. Thermodynamics—the physics of heat, work, and energy—is a tough subject, and it takes real chutzpah to jump in where many physicists fear to tread.

Although it may be difficult to grasp, thermodynamics is interesting. It has been described as the first revolutionary science. You probably don't really need it to study nutrition, but if you catch on to the basics, you will understand something that seems counterintuitive to many people. It will explain how you get more bang for your nutritional buck—that is, how you lose more weight per calorie.

When you consider that the fundamental unit in nutrition is the calorie, a unit of energy, it seems likely that it would be worth knowing something about the physics of energy exchange.

The Bottom Line on Metabolic Advantage

Here are the four main principles of metabolic advantage that will guide our discussion. The rest of the chapter will explain and justify these conclusions:

1. Metabolic advantage, or a better term, energy efficiency, is not contradicted by any physical law. Thermodynamics, in fact, more or less predicts variable energy efficiency. The way it has been discussed in nutrition is incorrect and does not conform to the way chemical thermodynamics is normally used.

2. Arguments against metabolic advantage often rely on practical considerations: how small the effect is. Yet the same critics espouse the value of cumulative small effects, operative in diets where you explicitly control calories, where 50 calories a day is supposed to add up over a year—and it doesn't. Metabolism doesn't work like that. Homeostatic (stabilizing) mechanisms compensate for simple changes in calories unless they are the right kind of calories, and in fact, the effects of different macronutrients can be dramatic. In any case, if there really is any change at all, that should be a call to figure out how to maximize that change, rather than ignore it.

3. Even if you aren't sure that metabolic advantage has been effectively demonstrated, it makes sense to try to make it work for you, since there is a great deal of potential scientific payoff.

4. Several mechanisms, particularly substrate cycling and gluconeogenesis, are involved. Experimentally, inefficiencies in digestion and metabolic processing (the so-called thermic effect of feeding) contribute as well.

Many people find metabolic advantage counterintuitive because the idea of energy conservation has been so deeply ingrained in their minds. I will explain the fallacy. I will present some of the data and then explain how the process plays out in terms of biochemical mechanisms.

The Data

There are basically two kinds of diet experiments. Some clearly show energy balance and some clearly do not. Here's an example of the former: If you take a normal person, keep them in a hospital room, and feed them constant calories (figure 9.1), you will find that it doesn't matter much how the calories are distributed among different foods. "Wide variations in the ratio of carbohydrate to fat do not alter total 24-h energy need"[2]—their weight will stay roughly constant. In some experimental cases, like this, a calorie is indeed just a calorie. Two people who are roughly similar in age and health will respond similarly to two isocaloric (same caloric value) diets regardless of the diet composition (amount of fat, carbohydrate, and protein). This means that, yes, calories count. Yet there are many exceptions.

The energy balance shown in figure 9.1 is achieved by biologic mechanisms, not the laws of thermodynamics. In those cases, where everything balances out, it isn't physical laws but rather the unique characteristics of

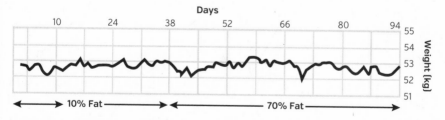

Figure 9.1. A thirteen-week study of a subject first on 10 percent (75 percent carbohydrate) of energy intake as fat and then on 70 percent (15 percent carbohydrate) of energy intake as fat. From J. Hirsch et al., "Diet Composition and Energy Balance in Humans," *American Journal of Clinical Nutrition* 67, no. 3 (1998): 551–55S.

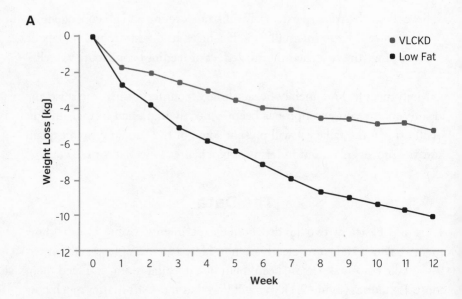

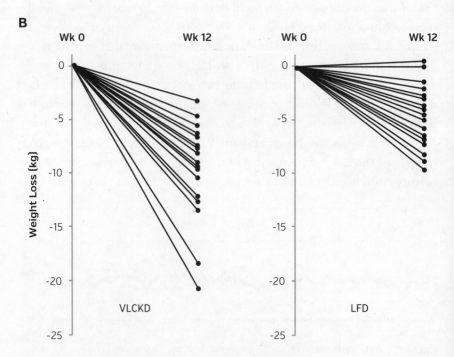

Figure 9.2. Comparison of low-carbohydrate ketogenic diet and low-fat diet. From J. S. Volek et al., "Carbohydrate Restriction Has a More Favorable Impact on the Metabolic Syndrome than a Low Fat Diet," *Lipids* 44, no. 4 (2009): 297–309.

living systems that keep things constant through the process of homeostasis. Big rule: In biology, almost everything is connected in feedback, and homeostatic mechanisms compensate for chemical changes. If you reduce your dietary intake of cholesterol, for example, your body will compensate by synthesizing new cholesterol. In view of this, the question we should be asking is, "How is energy balance possible when it is not predicted by thermodynamics?"; not, "How could there be different weight gain or loss for the same number of calories?" So let's look at the exceptions—the cases where the energy does not balance out—the second type of dietary experiment seen in the literature.

The exceptions can be dramatic. The experiment from the laboratory of Jeff Volek, then at the University of Connecticut, described previously in chapter 7, studied forty overweight men and women with metabolic syndrome (high triglycerides, low HDL, or at least two other factors). They were assigned to one of two ad libitum diets: a very low-carbohydrate ketogenic diet (VLCKD) (% carbohydrate [CHO]:fat:protein = 12:59:28), or a low-fat diet (%CHO:fat:protein = 56:24:20.) The experiment lasted twelve weeks. Although neither group was specifically told to reduce calories, both groups did show a spontaneous decrease in energy intake—it seems that if you sign up for a diet experiment, you automatically eat less.

Figure 9.2 shows the dramatic difference in performance between the VLCKD and the LFD. Figure 9.2*A* indicates the average effect: Weight loss in the VLCKD group was dramatically better. In reading the medical literature, however, it is important to ask about individual performance. People are different. Nobody loses an average amount of weight. People in both groups lost weight, but what is remarkable is the number of people on the VLCKD that lost *a lot of weight* (Figure 9.2*B*). Half of the people on the VLCKD lost more weight than the single most successful subject on the LFD.

Can You Trust Dietary Records?

Once again, there is the problem of patient dietary records. These records are known to be inaccurate, but not wildly so. Values can be off by 20 percent, but rarely by 50 percent, and are unlikely to be sole cause of the differences. Ketone bodies were measured, as well, so at least the VLCKD group did what they were told. It is important to reiterate that if the differences were due to inaccurate reporting of dietary intake (that is, if the diets were truly different in caloric intake), the people on the VLCKD must have overreported what they ate and the people on LFD must have underreported what they ate, or both. Bottom line: Food records have very high error rates. They are meaningful if the differences in the observed experimental differences are large, or if there are indicators of compliance such as the presence of ketone bodies.

Low-carbohydrate diets almost always win in a face-off with low-fat diets. Establishment nutritionists will write off the ties as wins, but they can only do so for so long. So if it is not just about the calories, where does thermodynamics really fit in? With the disclaimer of Sommerfeld's comments at the top of this chapter, I will give you a rough idea about how it's done in real biochemistry.

Thermodynamics

Thermodynamics is the physics of heat, work, and energy. The subject is simultaneously theoretical and mathematic, and fundamentally down to earth. Its roots are in the attempt to find out just how efficient a steam engine you can build. Thermodynamics came about during the industrial revolution, when the efficiency of steam engines was a big deal. In weight loss, we are really asking how efficiently food is utilized—much like the efficiency of a steam engine's fuel. The difficult side of thermodynamics is that its methods are highly mathematical and arcane, even for scientists. Thermodynamics has been described as "the science of partial differential equations," which is not to everybody's taste. The results, however, give you very simple equations for predicting things. It's a combination of heavy-duty theory and practical application. This is what those of us who are interested in thermodynamics actually like about it, and it's also the main theme of this book: Science with direct applicability. You get an equation that tells you whether you have a good steam engine, or, in fact, whether your food is fattening.

Real Thermodynamics

When people evoke the laws of thermodynamics, they're usually just talking about the first law, the law of conservation of energy. Unfortunately, "conservation of energy" has become a sound bite, at the level of "Einstein said that everything is relative." You have to know exactly what is being conserved, and more important, in thermodynamics, what is not. What follows is how thermodynamics is taught and used in science. The math is simple, but understanding depends on precise definitions and careful logic. What I'm about to cover many not be necessary for nutrition, but since thermodynamics is so often invoked, it is worth going through at least once.

The first law says precisely that there is a parameter called the internal energy and the change (Δ) in the internal energy of a system is equal to the heat, q, added to the system minus the work, w, that the system does on the environment. (The internal energy is usually written as U so as not to confuse it with the electrical potential.) In other words, the energy of a system is not determined directly, but rather by the difference between the heat and work that changes when the system changes.

$$\Delta U = q - w$$

This is how thermodynamics is taught. To get to the next step you need to understand the idea of a state variable. A state variable is a variable where any change is path-independent. For example, the familiar temperature, T, and pressure, P, are state variables: It doesn't matter whether you change the temperature quickly or slowly because the effect on the system is controlled only by the difference between the temperature after the change minus the temperature before the change (ΔT). The usual analogy is the as-the-crow-flies geographical distance, say, between New York and San Francisco. This is a state variable: It doesn't matter whether you fly directly or go through Memphis and Salt Lake City (like the flights I wind up on)—all that matters is the final state you arrive in.

The energy U is a state variable. Any process that you carry out will have a change in U that depends only on the initial and final states. However, q and w are NOT state variables (which is why they are written in lower case or with some other marking to distinguish them from state variables). How you design your machine will determine how much work you can get out of it and how much of the energy change will be wasted as heat. Looking at the biological case: Two different metabolic changes, such as responses to different meals, might have the same total energy change, but the work (both physical and chemical) and heat you generate are likely to differ if the two meals have very different inefficiencies. There is no theoretical reason why they couldn't have the same efficiency just by coincidence, but it is highly unlikely.

A preview of the second law is contained within the first law itself. The second law is what thermodynamics is really about—it is why thermodynamics took so long to evolve and why it is so hard to understand. The second law pretty much guarantees, contrary to popular misconception, that "a calorie is *not* a calorie."

Let's take a step back. There are four laws of thermodynamics, and the first law only operates in concert with the others. The zeroth law and the third law are pretty much theoretical, defining thermal equilibrium and the condition of absolute zero of temperature. It is the second law that embodies the special character of thermodynamics. Described by Ilya Prigogine, the Nobel prize–winning chemist and philosopher of thermodynamics, as the first revolutionary science, the second law explains how one diet can be more or less efficient that the other. The essential feature of the second law is the existence of a thing called entropy.

Entropy

Entropy is a measure of how disorganized a system is—that is, what its possibilities are. As described below, it is a measure of information. A gas filling a box completely is said to have higher entropy than a gas that is confined to only one side of the box. Another description: You would not need a very good GPS to find out if the molecule is in New York City versus whether it is in Yankee Stadium.

Entropy is traditionally defined with respect to a classic imaginary experiment. Although theoretical, it is clearly related to practical things. The experiment involves a creature referred to as the Maxwell's demon, who is capable of doing things perfectly smoothly and slowly without exerting any energy or creating any heat from friction. The experimental apparatus is a box with a partition—a membrane that separates the box into two compartments, one that is filled with a gas and one that is empty.

Maxwell's demon very carefully and slowly removes the membrane so that no work is done and no heat is generated. According to the first law of thermodynamics, which specifies the need to conserve energy and heat, nothing has really happened. In a real experiment, you could make an electronic device to open the partition so efficiently that it would hardly raise your electric bill—so effectively that energy is conserved and nothing should happen. Of course, you know that something will happen. The gas will fill up the whole box. Why? Because that's the way the world works according to the second law: Entropy will always increase and the gas will always spread as much as it can.

The gas fills up the whole box because it is the most probable way for the molecules to be distributed. The second law is about probability. Before the nineteenth century, physics held a view of a universe that was mechanical, a universe standing alone in time and controllable. The second law suddenly brought out the irreversible and statistical nature of things. It is not that nobody knew that time passed before that point, but the idea of physical processes running down like a clock—the notion of irreversible processes—was revolutionary. The history of physics shows how hard it is for people, even very smart people, to understand and cope with the idea of probability. As it evolved, however, the second law became very practical and explained how energy can be used to do work and how chemical reactions occur. It is the key to understanding energy transformation in life.

Entropy and Information

Entropy is about information. It is frequently said that increased entropy means increased disorder. The more precise way to put it would be that increased entropy means a less demanding way of arranging a system, and in turn, higher probability. In poker, a straight flush has much lower entropy than two of a kind because there are fewer ways to get a straight flush. Here's where it gets more complicated: Entropy—that is, information—can overpower energy. A receiver in American football can catch a pass even though he is double-teamed (his energy is compromised) because he has the information to know where the ball will be thrown. (The term *entropy* is also used in communications, where it indicates the extent to which a message has been corrupted during transmission.)

There are many ways to state the second law. One formal way says that it is impossible to carry out an operation where the sole effect is to transfer heat from a cold body to a warm body. This is obvious enough but it might not be easy to explain why. After all, the ocean is cold, but it has a huge amount of heat because it is so large. Why couldn't a ship extract a little bit of that heat to run its engines? That's the question Maxwell was really asking.

The original creature proposed by Maxwell was more sophisticated than the demon described above. This original demon sat on a membrane separating two compartments. One compartment had a hot gas, and the other, a cold gas. The partition had a little door—a very well-machined, well-oiled door, whose openings and closings did not require any real amount of work and did not generate any heat. The demon would look into the cold gas and if he saw a fast-moving particle, he would open the door and let the particle into the hot compartment. He would, similarly, let slow-moving particles move from the hot gas to the cold gas. The net effect was to transfer heat from a cold body to a warm body, a clear no-no according to the second law. It was a thought experiment, but you really could make a super efficient door, so why couldn't you make something at least close to this setup? The ocean is cold but it is so far from absolute zero and it is so big that there is so much heat, why couldn't you make something like a Maxwell's demon to get some of it to power your ocean liner? Was the second law not universal?

This paradox completely stumped physicists of the nineteenth century. It's because it's about probability and randomness and they were not used to thinking like that. The answer to Maxwell's paradox is that it is not really a paradox so much as another way of stating the second law. That's how the world is. Information costs. You can't make such a setup. If you could use some fancy electronic device to set up a sensor to distinguish between fast and slow molecules, it would still have to do work. The reason it gets confusing is that in the physical (real) world, we are only used to dealing with gross collections of things and averages. If we want to get down to single molecules, we have to run a machine to do it. The simpler way of saying it is that the reason that we can't make anything perfectly efficient is because we can't control individual molecules.

The point of all this is to say that, if you're going to carry out all the work, physical and chemical (that is, metabolic), using the energy from food, then you can't do it perfectly efficiently. Some part of the energy must be wasted. Of course, unlike an engineer, if you are trying to lose weight, the job of synthesizing and storing fat might be one that you want to run as inefficiently as possible.

The Second Law and Metabolic Advantage

There are many different ways of stating the second law, but one version emphasizes the fact that all real engines—in fact, all processes in the real world—are inherently inefficient—not just practically, not because you can't construct them so carefully that there's no friction, but theoretically, absolutely. There is no escape from inefficiency. The second law says that a perfect engine, living or otherwise, is not possible (unless you could get one to run at the mysterious temperature called absolute zero; the third law does give you that).

Inefficiency depends on where you stand and what you are trying to accomplish. In human beings, keeping warm (that is, using food for heat) might not be considered inefficient but from the point of view of a machine that is trying to manufacture protein and other cell material, it is energy that is wasted. The heat generated in the processing of food is called either thermic effect of feeding (TEF) or diet-induced thermogenesis (DIT). (The old name was "specific dynamic action.") These are a measure of energy wasted as heat. They are an expression of the inefficiency of the human machine. There are other ways to waste energy: for example, the so-called NEAT, nonexercise activity thermogenesis, which is the scientific name for fidgeting. The measured TEF of different macronutrients is different: Protein is much greater than carbohydrate, which is greater than fat. In other words, metabolic advantage is a well-documented fact, and the extent to which small changes add up is only a question of how you do the experiment. If you have to make glucose through the process of gluconeogenesis, rather than getting it from the diet, you are going to waste energy.

Beyond "Calories In = Calories Out"

In chemical thermodynamics we want to know whether a chemical reaction can be made to produce energy, or whether we have to put in energy to make the reaction go. As in the industrial revolution, we want to make an efficient chemical machine—we're thinking, of course, of a machine where you put in food and out comes enough energy to lift heavy weights, or more to the point, synthesize complicated chemicals like proteins. The key idea rests with identifying the likelihood of a reaction going forward with the reaction's ability to require or to give off energy. With the discussion of the second law behind us, we can guess that it is not about conservation. It is about dissipation of energy. The 4 kcal/g that we assign to the energy in carbohydrate is the energy exported from the reaction of oxidation to the environment. That's what you do in chemical thermodynamics. Otherwise, all food would have zero calories: The heat lost in oxidation is gained by the calorimeter. Calories in equals calories out, sure, but that literally leaves you with absolutely nothing.

What comes next shows you how real thermodynamics works. It is not particularly mathematical. All you need is high school algebra. You can see the beauty of thermodynamics and how it can tell you, right off, that it's not just calories in, calories out (commonly abbreviated CICO on social media). You may like it, but if you prefer to avoid the math, you can skip to the summary at the end.

The second law says, in essence, that all (real) systems are inefficient. In practice, the law can be used to tell you whether a chemical reaction actually produces energy or, as we have said, whether you will have to put in energy to make it go. This is the key in chemistry (and living systems in general): Does the reaction proceed as written?

When we write A → B, we want to know whether the reaction will proceed from left to right spontaneously. "Spontaneously" means without the addition of energy. It does not mean fast, which is a separate question. The 4 kcal of energy that you measure in the calorimeter is both a measure of the tendency of the reaction to occur (oxidations generally go easily by themselves and produce energy) and also the maximum energy available to do work. They are very closely related, because although living systems do mechanical work, the main use of the energy is in chemical work: synthesizing metabolites and cell material. The second law leads to the definition of a number of different forms of the energy that are used under different conditions. The particular form of the energy that is used under conditions of constant temperature and pressure—the conditions in which biochemists typically work—is called the Gibbs free energy, which is almost always abbreviated with the letter G, and whose change is written with the Greek delta, ΔG. The Gibbs free energy for a chemical is precisely defined as the maximum work you can get from running the reaction at constant temperature and pressure, and it is identified with the tendency of the reaction to go in the forward direction. The 4 kcal produced by the oxidation of glucose tells you that is the most you could get out of it in terms of work or driving other chemical reactions. In practice, some energy might be wasted as heat or other unproductive processes.

To summarize what we have just discussed: Chemical thermodynamics emphasizes the reaction of the system, not the whole universe. We want to know about the energy exchange when we burn food. The complete oxidation of glucose in the calorimeter produces 4 kcal. It is not about conservation. It is about dissipation of energy.

The word *thermodynamics* is thrown around a lot in nutrition, mostly by people who have no idea what it's about. Again, you don't need thermodynamics to do nutrition, but if you're going to bring thermodynamics into the picture, you have to do it right. So, in case you want to see what people really do in chemical thermodynamics, I will present a good example.

Let's begin with energy change, meaning Gibbs free energy. Here we have a grand rule: If the free energy change is negative ($\Delta G < 0$) for the reaction, the reaction is downhill, will go by itself, and will give off energy (which you might be able to capture by coupling it to another chemical reaction or to some mechanical, electrical, or heat machine). The Gibbs free energy has two components, the heat of reaction, called enthalpy (ΔH) and the entropy (ΔS).

Here's a simple example of what you might do in real thermodynamics, which will also illustrate why the calorie equivalence idea in nutrition is not right. Suppose that you wanted to know about the formation of carbon monoxide (CO)—if carbon is oxidized to CO, how much energy is given off in the process. Generally thought of in the context of a poison, CO has other uses—small amounts are actually produced in the human body. So, we want to know: Is the oxidation of carbon to CO uphill or downhill and by how much? To keep it simple, we'll take the enthalpy (heat of reaction, ΔH). We can do the experiment so that the entropy is not an important player (low temperature). The heat of reaction is easily measured.

In the case of oxidizing carbon, then, if heat is given off ($\Delta H = (-)$), the reaction will be spontaneous and go by itself. The problem with trying to figure out how much energy you can get by burning carbon to carbon monoxide is that you can't really measure it. If you try to carry out the reaction, you always get some CO_2. So, what can you do? Here's how to deal with it: We can't measure the heat of reaction for oxidation of carbon to CO directly (again, because it is always complicated by some CO_2 being formed), but we can measure the enthalpy of burning of carbon to CO_2 (a minus sign means heat is given off):

$$C + O_2 \rightarrow CO_2 \quad \Delta H = -94 \text{ kcal}$$

We also know the energy of burning CO to CO_2:

$$CO + \tfrac{1}{2} O_2 \rightarrow CO_2 \quad \Delta H = -68 \text{ kcal}$$

Another great simplifying feature of thermodynamics is that if we know the energy for a chemical reaction (or any process), the energy for going the other way is the same numerically, only with the opposite sign, so:

$$CO_2 \rightarrow CO + \tfrac{1}{2} O_2 \quad \Delta H = +68 \text{ kcal}$$

The energy functions, G and H, are state functions. Remember from earlier in this chapter that means they are path-independent, or independent of the conditions under which a particular reaction is carried. State functions can be added just as in simple algebra. The energies add up (figure 9.3). Here you see the beauty of thermodynamics. The attraction to those of us who like it is that you can manipulate the results with elementary algebra. The great simplicity in this kind of calculation reflects its highly predictive power.

What did we do? We had two different paths from carbon to carbon monoxide: one (two-step) path that we could calculate, and one that we are trying to find out. We knew they must be equal. The principle that allows you to add up heats of reaction is called Hess's Law.

Hess's Law Shows That a Calorie Is Not a Calorie

The idea that "a calorie is a calorie," means that the energy yield for metabolism will be path-independent—that is, the same for all diets and

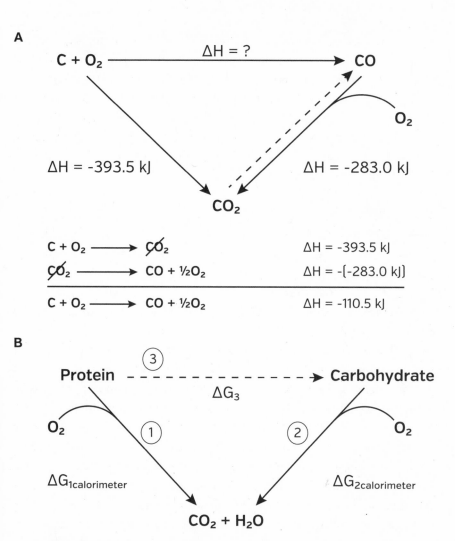

Figure 9.3. Hess's Law. *A*, Calculating heat of reaction for formation of CO. Path of the arrows (measured) must equal the direct conversion to CO, so we just add them up. *B*, According to Hess's Law (adding up energies), the energy for path 1, ΔG_1 should be equal to the energy for path 3 followed by path 2, $\Delta G_1 - \Delta G_2$. Using calorimeter values and the principle that a calorie is a calorie leads to a contradiction. *Note:* Energies in figure in kJ = 4.28 kcal.

proportional to the calorimeter values. To show that this is not true in general we use the simple additive property of state variables as in the carbon monoxide problem above. We will look at oxidation of protein by two pathways, either directly, or indirectly by first converting the protein to glucose through gluconeogenesis (GNG) and then oxidizing the glucose to CO_2. The laws of thermodynamics say that these should be the same.

The calorimeter values say that energy yield for carbohydrate and for protein are equivalent: ΔG (oxidation) = -4 kcal/mol (figure 9.2). The (-) sign, again, means energy is given off and the process is spontaneous. Here's the plan. We make multiple paths for oxidizing protein: path 1 (direct), and paths 2 and 3 (indirect):

Path 1: Protein + O_2 $\rightarrow$ CO_2 + H_2O ΔG_1 = 4 kcal/g

Path 2: Carbohydrate + O_2 $\rightarrow$ CO_2 + H_2O ΔG_2 = 4 kcal/g

Path 3: Protein—GNC $\rightarrow$ Carbohydrate + O_2 $\rightarrow$ CO_2 + H_2O ΔG_3 + ΔG_2 = ?

In path 1, we burn protein directly to CO_2. Because free energy is a state variable, the free energy ΔG_1 must be equal to the sum of ΔG_2, the energy for path 2, plus ΔG_3, the energy for path 3. This means that ΔG_3 for path 3 must be about zero. However, path 3 includes the process of gluconeogenesis. Chemistry students work very hard in order to learn that gluconeogenesis is an expensive, endergonic (energy requiring) process: It costs energy (about 6 ATP) to turn a mole of protein into a mole of carbohydrate. It is the failure to take this into account—the assumption that only the calories measured in a calorimeter are important—that leads to a contradiction. Once you take into account the real metabolic processes, it becomes clear that "a calorie is a calorie" is not a valid principle. The example bears on the real behavior of living systems, and is likely a contributor to the benefits of dietary carbohydrate restriction. More generally, if one diet is reported to be more effective for weight loss than another, there is no reason not to take it seriously. Like any scientific result, it should be evaluated carefully, but if it is your body mass that you are concerned about, the stakes are high.

The Nonequilibrium Picture

There is one more level of sophistication to address. To some extent, it is not really about thermodynamics at all, or at least not equilibrium thermodynamics (the energy required to go between states in equilibrium).

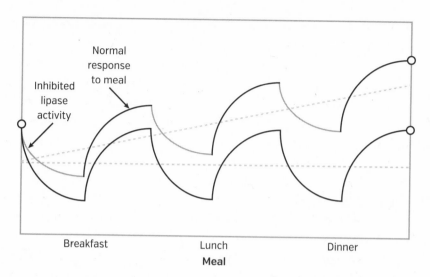

Figure 9.4. Hypothetical model for the effect of insulin on efficiency of storage. The lower line, indicating response under conditions of weight maintenance, fluctuates but averages to no change. The upper line shows the effect of added insulin on hormone-sensitive lipase activity. The important point is that the energy differences are very small compared to the equilibrium value, which would be very far below the figure. The system is not controlled by energy but by rates.

Equilibrium thermodynamics is what is usually studied, and we are taught that rates of reaction are considered separately from energy. Equilibrium thermodynamics tell, for example, that amino acids are more stable than proteins. The rate of breakdown is very slow. If you could keep the bacteria off your steak it would last for months, or even years, but at the end of time it would be all amino acids, (or even simpler things). In biochemistry, however, rates become important because living systems are not at equilibrium until they die. Things are moving forward. All the reactions in biology are run by catalysts—that is, enzymes that control the speed of a reaction, rather than the energetics. A better way to put it might be to say that the key players in all this are hormones and hormones generally affect enzymes, which in turn affect rates, not energy.

Living systems are not at equilibrium. Living systems, in fact, maintain themselves very far from equilibrium. They are characterized by an in-and-out flux of material and energy. In a dietary intervention, material fluctuates around a level far from equilibrium. In other words, changes with time become important and changes might be controlled by the presence of catalysts—enzymes or other factors that affect the rate of reaction.

Figure 9.4 shows the theoretical fluctuations of fat within a fat cell. The key idea is that the reactions, breakdown, and resynthesis of the fat molecule are very far from equilibrium (at equilibrium, you would have very little fat, mostly fatty acid, and free glycerol). Looking at fat gain and loss (figure 9.4), adipocytes cycle between states of greater or lesser net breakdown of fat (lipolysis and reformation) depending on the hormonal state, which in turn is dependent on the macronutrient composition of the diet. A hypothetical scheme for changes in adipocyte TAG and a proposal for how TAG gain or loss could be different for isocaloric diets with different levels of insulin is shown in the figure. The basic idea is that fat fluctuates, but if you slowly store enough so that the fat molecules you form don't have a chance to break down before you consume another meal, fat will accumulate regardless of caloric input.

Under normal control conditions of weight maintenance, the breakdown and utilization of TAG follows a pattern of lipolysis (fasting), and intake plus resynthesis (meals). To make it simple, let's assume a sudden, instantaneous spike in food at meals. Then the curves represent the net flow of material within the adipocyte. This averages out to a stable weight maintenance (lower dotted line in figure 9.4). If we keep each meal at constant calories but increase the percentage of carbohydrate or otherwise generate a higher insulin level, the hormone-sensitive lipases, the enzymes that catalyze the breakdown of fat, will be inhibited (the solid line in figure 9.4). Resynthesis of TAG is thus less affected by the elevated insulin and might actually slow down. The net effects are changes in the direction of accumulation of TAG. It is theoretical, but the model shows you how kinetics (how fast things happen) might be more important than thermodynamics (how stable they are at the end of the reaction).

PART 3

The Low-Carbohydrate Diet for Disease

CHAPTER 10

Diabetes

At the end of our clinic day, we go home thinking, "The clinical improvements are so large and obvious, why don't other doctors understand?" Carbohydrate-restriction is easily grasped by patients: because carbohydrates in the diet raise the blood glucose, and as diabetes is defined by high blood glucose, it makes sense to lower the carbohydrate in the diet. By reducing the carbohydrate in the diet, we have been able to taper patients off as much as 150 units of insulin per day in 8 days, with marked improvement in glycemic control—even normalization of glycemic parameters.

—ERIC WESTMAN[1]

The scene is lunch in the cafeteria at SUNY Downstate Medical Center. I am going on about how strange it is that carbohydrate is recommended for people with diabetes, a disease whose most salient symptom is high blood glucose. Overhearing my story, several clinicians at the table ask incredulously, almost in unison, "Who gives carbohydrates to diabetics?" I say, "The American Diabetes Association (ADA). They recommend 55–60 percent carbs (or whatever their values were at the time)." Their response? I believe the cliché is "deafening silence." It's true. The ADA recommends high-carbohydrate diets to be compensated for with medication. Sugar is okay as long as you "cover with insulin." That was really their recommendation, at least in 2010: "Sucrose-containing foods can be substituted for other carbohydrates in the meal plan or, if added to the meal plan, covered with insulin or other glucose lowering medications." In 2013 they finally, and quite quietly, dropped this bizarre and ultimately harmful recommendation, but it remains a testament to their willingness to recommend a dietary treatment that will make things worse so that more drugs can be taken, or more accurately, *because* more drugs can be taken.

The folks at the table were not endocrinologists and they were of my generation. They grew up knowing that you don't give carbohydrates to people with diabetes. Simple. After all, it will increase their blood sugar, which is precisely what you are trying to prevent in those who have the disease. Because it was not their medical specialization, the clinicians were unaware that recommendations had evolved at official agencies, or even that it is now politically incorrect to refer to patients as "diabetics" (unless you yourself are a person with diabetes). They believed in the old common-sense idea that because diabetes was a disease of carbohydrate intolerance, cutting out carbohydrate should be the first line of attack—and they probably knew that it worked. Why wouldn't it work?

Diabetes: Type 1 and Type 2

Diabetes is a disease—several diseases, really—of carbohydrate intolerance. In type 1 the intolerance is due to the inability of the pancreas to produce insulin in response to carbohydrate, and in type 2 it is due to poor cellular response to the insulin that is produced, accompanied by deterioration of the insulin-producing cells of the pancreas. The most salient symptom of diabetes (and a major contributor to the pathology) is high blood sugar, which, not surprisingly, is most effectively treated by reducing dietary carbohydrates. The common clinical measurements are: (1) fasting blood glucose (sometimes written FBG), usually given in units of milligrams per deciliter (mg/dL) and normal considered to be around 100 mg/dL; (2) an oral glucose tolerance test (sometimes abbreviated OGTT), the response in the blood to a dose of glucose; and (3) the percent of hemoglobin A1c (HbA1c), a modified form of hemoglobin (that has reacted with blood glucose) that is a measure of the cumulative effect of the high blood sugar. Normal levels for the latter are about 5 percent, but people with diabetes can have values of 20 percent. In type 1, patients are required to inject insulin, whereas people with type 2 are advised to improve their lifestyle "with diet and exercise." If those with type 2 cannot lower their blood sugar with diet—the diet that their doctor recommends is unlikely to adequately do so—they will also require insulin or other drugs for reduction of glucose, of which there are many. The insulin level of 150 units per day cited in the introductory quotation to this chapter is a very high dose. Coming off such a high dose is a major accomplishment, suggesting that Eric Westman's diet might be better than the standard, and of course, reduction in medication is considered improvement in all the diseases that I know of.

Why Diabetes?

Diabetes stands at the forefront of the nutrition problem because it's so clearly linked to control of metabolism and the glucose–insulin axis. Correspondingly, it shows exactly what carbohydrate restriction can do for you. Diabetes is, in a real sense, the extreme version of the nutritional problem in obesity and possibly heart disease. Although Atkins or other low-carbohydrate diets are used as a therapy for overweight or obesity, they are not just about weight loss. In fact, they are not even primarily about weight loss, despite the fact that they are more frequently used by people who are overweight than by those with diabetes. Many diets work for weight loss, and calorie restriction may or may not be part of the reason that a low-carbohydrate diet makes you lose weight, but to bring diabetes under control, we know that you have to reduce carbohydrate regardless of whether or not calories go down, and regardless of whether or not you lose weight.

The intuitive idea that people with diabetes should not consume much sugar or starch is a good principle. Nothing in the science contradicts this. However effective a diet is for treatment, nobody really knows what is required for prevention because it is often a kind of hidden disease. Early symptoms might be low-level, such as simple irritability and fatigue, and type 2, in particular, can have a very slow onset. As a treatment, however, a low-carbohydrate diet is better than drugs for most people. This is knowledge we cannot afford to ignore, considering how terrible a disease diabetes is: It is the major cause of acquired blindness and the major cause of amputations after accidents.

Where Does It Come From?

In chapter 5, I described Claude Bernard's revolutionary discovery of the liver's control of blood glucose and its regulation of glycogen turnover and gluconeogenesis (GNG). Bernard voiced astonishment at finding sugar in a dog that hadn't consumed any sugar. Historians suspect, however, that writing about it later he might have exaggerated how much the original observations really took him by surprise. He wouldn't be the first and undoubtedly will not be the last scientist to revise the history of his discoveries for dramatic effect. It makes for a great story to have the answer fall from heaven, especially if you can describe the intervention of your prepared mind, as Pasteur put it.

It is likely that Claude Bernard had suspected for a long time that animals could make their own sugar. He guessed that it could be made from fat—which was not true—or from protein—which was true. One clue that would have led him in this direction was his observation that people with diabetes had more glucose in their blood than could be accounted for by dietary intake alone. He must have suspected that those people with diabetes were making their own sugar. In fact, gluconeogenesis goes on all the time in the body, whether or not you have diabetes. GNG is not, as the textbooks sometimes imply, a last-ditch resource during starvation, after glycogen is depleted.

GNG goes on all the time. As described in chapter 5, when you wake up in the morning, half of your blood glucose might come from GNG. The difference for people with diabetes is that they have lost the ability to turn it off at the right time. This is due to the reduction or absence of insulin, as in type 1, or the poor response to the insulin that occurs in type 2. In healthy individuals, the presence of glucose coming in from the diet causes insulin secretion, which then inhibits gluconeogenesis and glycogen breakdown. Many people think that the high blood sugar seen in diabetes is due to a failure in clearance because the cells cannot take up the glucose in the blood for fuel. Even the textbooks make this claim. While the number of GLUT4 receptors in people with diabetes does not increase in response to dietary glucose as much as it does in healthy people, it seems that this is not the major cause of hyperglycemia—people with diabetes still have enough of these glucose-transporting receptors under most conditions.

The major problem, in fact, appears to be the persistence of glucose production from the liver. Under normal conditions, release of glucose from liver glycogen and gluconeogenesis are both regulated by insulin and glucagon. As glucose goes up, insulin goes up and glucagon goes down. In response, the liver stops producing additional glucose. A key feature of diabetes is the loss of this stimulus-response control over glucose production. With that in mind, it does not make sense to recommend dietary glucose to people with diabetes, as it will simply sit on top of the unregulated level of built-in production.

Can You Treat It?

Dietary carbohydrate restriction has been a therapy for diabetes since before the discovery of insulin.[2] It is not a new idea that blood glucose control has positive effects on all of the downstream effects of the disease, including lipid markers for, and incidence of, cardiovascular disease. For many diabetes sufferers, dietary carbohydrate restriction is all that is needed to improve or eliminate symptoms. Normal glucose control, stable weight, and normal lipids can be attained, and the benefits persist as long as carbohydrate intake is low. It then becomes a semantic question whether someone can be called "cured" if they have to stay on a prescribed diet indefinitely. The real question is whether a low-carbohydrate diet, or the high-carbohydrate diet recommended by health agencies, the one that was associated with onset of the diabetes, is the more extreme.

A key issue is the established association between body weight and type 2 diabetes, and whether the association is causal. Studies by researchers at the University of Minnesota provide strong evidence against the idea that there is a causal link between the two. Nuttall and Gannon have produced a series of well-designed, well-controlled experiments demonstrating the value of carbohydrate restriction in treating diabetes under conditions where no weight is lost. They found that carbohydrate restriction has a consistent and dramatic ability to reduce high blood glucose, even when there is no change in body mass. It is not easy to lose weight, so the ability to treat diabetes without concern for weight loss provides an obvious advantage. From a theoretical standpoint, Nuttall and Gannon's studies support the idea that both obesity and diabetes are reflections of a central cause—disruptions in the glucose–insulin axis, most likely. In other words, obesity and diabetes might stand in a parallel, rather than serial, relation to each other. The most obvious evidence to support this idea is the fact that there are people with diabetes, both types 1 and 2, who are not fat, and of course, most fat people do not have diabetes.

The obstinate refusal of endocrinologists and diabetes educators to face these ideas, and hardest to understand, their reluctance to face Nuttall and Gannon's experimental results, remains a major obstacle in dealing with the current epidemic. Almost every statement, whether from health agencies or individual experts, continues to emphasize weight loss as the prime goal of diabetes treatment, and endocrinologists continue to make this their recommendation. The problem is that the scientific evidence on the subject is just not on their radar. Why not? Endocrinologists already have to retain so much medical knowledge that it's not entirely surprising that they don't know much about nutrition. There is no excuse, however, for the endocrinologists who act as if they know nutrition but refuse to consider low-carbohydrate diets. I doubt that they love their patients any less, but perhaps they love hating Dr. Atkins more.

Low-GI versus Real Low-Carbohydrate

If low–GI is good, how about no–GI?

—ERIC WESTMAN

In 2008, David Jenkins compared a diet high in cereal with a low–glycemic index diet.[3] As I explained in chapter 2, the glycemic index is a measure of the actual effect of dietary glucose on blood glucose. Pioneered by Jenkins and coworkers, a low-GI diet is based on the same rationale as a low-carbohydrate diet: that glycemic and insulin fluctuations pose a metabolic risk. GI emphasizes "the type of carbohydrate," thus offering a politically correct form of low-carbohydrate diet. As stated in the 2008 study:

> We selected a high cereal fiber diet treatment for its *suggested health benefits* for the comparison so that the *potential value of carbohydrate foods* could be emphasized equally for both high cereal fiber and low–glycemic index interventions. (Emphasis added)

After the completion of the twenty-four-week study Jenkins concluded: "In patients with type 2 diabetes, 6-month treatment with a low–glycemic index diet resulted in moderately lower HbA1c levels compared with a high–cereal fiber diet." Coincidentally, on almost the same day that David Jenkins's study came out, Eric Westman's group published a study that compared a low-GI diet with a true low-carbohydrate diet.[4] The studies were comparable in duration and number of subjects, and a direct comparison (figure 10.1) shows that the true low-carbohydrate has much greater benefits—hence the quotation from Dr. Westman at the head of this section.

Figure 10.1 by itself constitutes the best evidence for a low-carbohydrate diet as the "default diet," the one to try first, for diabetes and metabolic

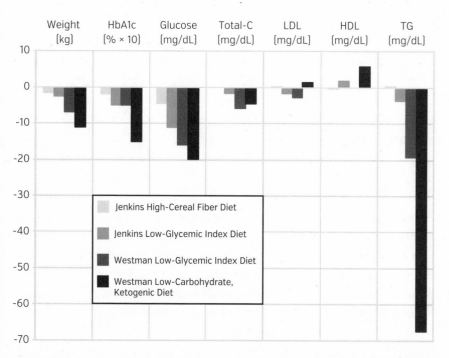

Figure 10.1. Effect of high–cereal fiber or low–glycemic index diets on body weight and hHbA1c. Data from D. J. Jenkins et al., "Effect of a Low-Glycemic Index or a High-Cereal Fiber Diet on Type 2 Diabetes: A Randomized Trial," *Journal of the American Medical Association* 300, no. 23 (2008): 2742–2753; E. C. Westman et al., "The Effect of a Low-Carbohydrate, Ketogenic Diet Versus a Low-Glycemic Index Diet on Glycemic Control in Type 2 Diabetes Mellitus," *Nutrition and Metabolism* 5, no. 36 (2008).

syndrome. There are hundreds of studies about all aspects of diabetes but none contradict the benefits of carbohydrate reduction shown in figure 10.1. It is worth noting, however, that one additional benefit wasn't addressed by Westman's study: Low-carbohydrate diet reliably reduces the dependence on drugs. In William Yancy's classic study[5] of twenty-one patients on low-carbohydrate ketogenic diets, all but four reduced their level of medication and seven patients discontinued medication altogether. Reducing medication, in and of itself, is a huge advance. Is that it? That's it. The hundreds of papers published provide a variety of details about this very complicated disease and its response to the numerous drugs that are used as therapy, but the basic principles described here have never been refuted in any fundamental way.

Diabetes is a central battleground in the new low-carbohydrate revolution and it is likely to provide a major victory. Scientifically, the burden of proof is on those who continue to claim that it is a good idea for people with diabetes to consume any significant amount of carbohydrate. Impressive as the comparison shown in figure 10.1 is, it has made little impact. Establishment medicine has arbitrarily decided that long-term randomized controlled trials (RCTs) are a kind of "gold standard." Whatever their value for particular types of experiments, this principle is used to ignore any other type of study, especially if it challenges the party line. RCT studies can be useful, but the people who insist on using them for diabetes sit on panels that would never fund an RCT study if it included low-carbohydrate diets. Moreover, an RCT is not the best thing for everything. It is one kind of experiment, and all possibilities are not up for grabs in science. Since diabetes is primarily about carbohydrate, there is no better treatment than reducing carbohydrate. There is nothing in the outcome of low-carbohydrate trials of whatever length to suggest harm from such a therapeutic regimen—only benefit. Absolute dependence on arbitrary rules and "gold standards" is what continues to cause the most harm.

What About Cardiovascular Disease?

The "concerns" about low-carbohydrate diets still revolve around the imagined risk of cardiovascular disease from fat in the diet despite the continued failure to show any such risk. Carbohydrate restriction actually improves the usual markers of CVD—notably, HDL ("good cholesterol") and triglycerides. Although there haven't yet been long-term trials to show that carbohydrate reduction prevents CVD, there are plenty of long-term trials on the effect of reducing fat, and they all fail to show any clinically significant effect.

There is a strong association between diabetes and the incidence of CVD, but the largely discredited, or at least greatly exaggerated, diet–heart hypothesis—and its proscriptions against dietary fat—has caused us to ignore the carbohydrate elephant in the room. It turns out, however, that the best predictor of microvascular complications (blindness, amputations) and, to a lesser extent, macrovascular complications (heart attack, stroke) in patients with type 2 diabetes is hemoglobin A1c, which is under the control of chronic dietary carbohydrate consumption. Data from the United Kingdom Prevention of Diabetes Study (UKPDS)[6] provide support for this idea. In some sense, increased risk of CVD for people with diabetes is due simply to the diabetes itself. More precisely, the same conditions that gave rise to the diabetic state—disruptions in the glucose–insulin axis—increase the risk of vascular disease.

Summary

Diabetes is a disease of carbohydrate intolerance. Type 1 is characterized by an inability to produce insulin in response to carbohydrate, and in type 2, there is peripheral insulin resistance along with deterioration of the beta cells of the pancreas. The most salient symptom of diabetes (and a major contributor to the pathology) is high blood sugar, which, not surprisingly, is most effectively treated by reducing dietary carbohydrates. The clinical measurements are: (1) fasting blood glucose; (2) an oral glucose tolerance test, the response in the blood to a dose of glucose; and (3) the percent of modified hemoglobin, hemoglobin A1c (HbA1c). It is not hard to guess the best treatment for a disease characterized by poor response to ingested carbohydrates, but you do need to know if the theory will hold up in practice. A personal story might bring this into perspective.

Wendy's Story

The Uses of Metabolic Adversity

By Wendy Pogozelski

Wendy Pogozelski is professor and chairman of biochemistry at SUNY Geneseo in upstate New York. One of the people who has used low-carbohydrate diets to teach metabolism, she developed type 1 diabetes as an adult. In 2012, ASBMB Today, *the house organ of the American Society of Biochemistry and Molecular Biology, started a series about challenges to biochemists. Wendy's story was their first publication in this series:*

Blurred vision was the first sign that something was wrong. The front row of the freshman chemistry class I was teaching looked strangely fuzzy. Then, over the next few days, I was gripped by an unquenchable thirst and was constantly fatigued. Seemingly overnight I lost eight pounds. I recognized the symptoms of diabetes, but I was young(ish), slim(ish) and an avid kickboxer. Mine was not the typical diabetic profile.

Despite my suspicion that I was experiencing raging hyperglycemia, the diagnosis—"You have diabetes"—was devastating. It marked the beginning of a lifestyle that is an enormous challenge. However, the journey has led me to an increased understanding of biochemistry, has enhanced my teaching and ultimately has cast me in a new role of helping others. It turned out that I had developed latent autoimmune diabetes in adults, or LADA, a subset of type 1 diabetes. LADA is due to an autoimmune reaction to pancreatic glutamate decarboxylase, or GAD65. While LADA has a slower onset than classic type 1, formerly known as juvenile diabetes, the two diseases follow a similar course and require injections of insulin.

Fortunately, I felt equipped to manage my condition. I teach metabolism to undergraduates using an approach that emphasizes insulin-dependent pathways as a unifying theme and one that offers an everyday context. I knew that carbohydrates, whether whole grain or highly processed, could raise my blood glucose to dangerous levels, so my response to the diagnosis was to reduce greatly carbohydrates in my diet. In addition, I was careful to monitor my blood sugar levels and insulin doses. The result was that my hemoglobin A1c (glycosylated hemoglobin, a measure of blood sugar control) was 5.4 percent, within the normal 4 percent to 5 percent range. My doctor said that I was his "best patient ever" and that I was achieving the blood sugars of a nondiabetic person.

Despite satisfaction with my glycemic control, my physician wanted me to see a dietitian. To my surprise, the dietitian was appalled by my diet. She said, "You have to eat a minimum of 130 grams of carbohydrates a day." I protested, but she recruited the rest of the medical team to endorse her position: "We all say you have to eat more carbs. The American Diabetes Association gives us these guidelines." One member of the team said, "I want you to eat chocolate. I want you to enjoy life."

As someone raised to be cooperative, and because I found it easy to embrace medical advice to eat chocolate, I agreed to eat more carbohydrates. The result was that my HbA1c rose above 7 percent. My blood sugar levels were frequently in the 200 to 300 mg/dL range (far above the normal level of about 85 mg/dL), even when I supplemented with extra insulin. My former dose of seven units of insulin per day increased to 30 units per day. The loss of control was immensely frustrating. My physician attributed my initial success to what is called the diabetes honeymoon. Often, when someone first begins taking insulin, there is a short-lived period during which beta cells seem to recover a bit and secrete insulin. Regardless, it was clear that the dietitian's approach was not yielding the success I desired. I felt confused and uncertain as to what to do.

I decided to investigate for myself what my best diet should be. I studied the literature, I sought out researchers and physicians, and I attended countless metabolism-related talks. In addition, I connected with hundreds of people with diabetes. The most important contribution to my achieving clarity, however, was evaluating literature based on a molecular understanding of how metabolism works.

In my quest for answers, I found to my surprise that many dietitians and physicians were unable to explain the basis for the dietary recommendations they endorsed. Some did, however, express a desire for a better understanding or review of what they'd once learned. And in the general public, I encountered scores of diabetics and nondiabetics who also wanted tools to make sense of conflicting nutritional information.

I began to use what I had learned not only to expand and improve my teaching and research but also to step into the role of a nutrition explainer. First I was determined to see that none of my students would lack understanding of processes such as gluconeogenesis and the many pathways affected by insulin. I created new lecture topics and problem sets based on diabetes and nutrition applications. My students responded positively and appreciatively. There was a palpable increase in attention in class.

Students came to my office to chat about things that they had read. My class evaluations praised the use of nutritional context and often said, "This material could have been rather dull without all these great applications." I even heard (frequently) "I love metabolism!"

Beyond my student population, I engaged a world of bloggers, physicians and other people with diabetes, many of whom were eager to understand more deeply how things work metabolically. I now find myself being interviewed, quoted in papers, and invited to speak to groups of people, including physicians, who want to deepen their understanding of metabolic pathways. I am asked to share my nutrition-based teaching applications with other professors and with textbook publishers. In these efforts, I try to avoid dispensing nutritional advice; instead, I attempt to show how nutrient composition affects metabolic pathways so that my audience feels better able to evaluate nutritional recommendations.

Five years later, diabetes is still an immense mental and physical challenge, but I am grateful for the insight and tools that my education and training have provided me. Most importantly, if I am able to further the use of molecular science to help others find optimal dietary strategies, and if I can help the next generation, then my adversity will have had a positive outcome.

Epilogue

The story in *ASBMB Today* was written for a series on how scientists overcome hard times rather than as a treatise on how to manage diabetes. However, the essay was read by many folks who were interested from a standpoint of their own health concerns. I received many requests for an update, as people wondered if, after my foray into inclusion of carbohydrates, I returned to my low-carbohydrate style of eating. The answer is a resounding "yes." (With one small caveat, as you'll see below.)

As I studied the scientific literature, I became more and more convinced that my absolute primary concern should be keeping my blood sugar levels as close to normal as possible. I saw that I achieve the flattest blood sugars when I keep my carbohydrate low and my insulin low. Dr. Richard Bernstein, a type 1 diabetic and engineer-turned-physician who pioneered the use of glucose meters, calls this principle "the law of small numbers."

Carbohydrate restriction results in minimization of errors. Hyperglycemia and hypoglycemia come from mis-estimation of carbohydrate amount, rate of carbohydrate absorption and insulin absorption and activity. These factors are nearly impossible to predict accurately. Many people who use large amounts of insulin to cover large amounts of carbohydrate in their diet frequently find themselves in dangerous situations (passing out, etc.) when the peak activity of the insulin occurs earlier than the peak absorption of the dietary carbohydrate. I have never passed out and my health care team has been astounded by my lack of hypoglycemic episodes. Hyperglycemia also needs to be avoided though. It is these high blood sugars that correlate with the long-term deleterious effects of diabetes. Observing the diabetic amputees at the endocrinologist's office and watching people painfully shuffle into the dialysis center has been strong motivation to avoid these high blood sugars.

What is the evidence for the effectiveness of a low-carb dietary approach with me? I was used as a test subject for "sensor" technology. This device consists of a needle, sensor and a transmitter worn on the body and it communicates with an insulin pump. When my results were printed out after the experiment, my health care team was astonished at how level my glucose readings were. I was the last appointment of the day and all the workers gathered around to admire the printout of the "beautiful" blood sugars and ask me how in the world I did that. (This was at the office where the team had insisted that I needed to eat carbohydrate. Yes, it was very satisfying.)

It is worth noting too how well having level blood sugar makes me feel. When my blood sugar goes over 200 mg/dL, I start to feel melodramatic and have an elevated emotional response to even minor difficulties. Low blood sugar induces glucagon and epinephrine hormone release, which result in sweating and a feeling of panic as well as low energy. Both high and low blood sugar make my brain sluggish. Also, as a headache-prone person for much of my life, I found that my formerly frequent headaches nearly disappeared when I began to practice carbohydrate restriction.

When I keep my meal at less than 10 g of carbohydrate, my blood sugars rise by no more than 40 mg/dL; sometimes they rise as little as 10 mg/dL, but regardless, they return to normal within two hours—like a nondiabetic. I find that too much protein will elevate my blood sugar so I keep that amount moderate but I don't consciously restrict it, or my fat.

Despite my knowledge that carbohydrate restriction is best for me, I sometimes have deviated from this plan of attack. Particularly, since I became a mom, there has been a lot more carbohydrate in the kitchen tempting me. Couple that with the chronic exhaustion of motherhood and you've got a situation that makes reaching for carbohydrate much more likely. I rediscovered that M&Ms (used effectively for potty-training a toddler) are delicious, and my plans to eat no more than three have consistently been shown to be no match for whatever else is at work. (My theory is that there is an evil force activated when one eats M&Ms and he is only appeased when the bag is empty.) Every time I have indulged, however, I have always concluded "It wasn't worth it" when I saw my high blood sugars or had to compensate for my over-estimation of my insulin.

I also decided that I really, really like dark chocolate and given that it is full of antioxidants, I do allow myself some. I save my carbs for it. The 85% variety I eat has 4 g/square and is much more satisfying than milk chocolate, so it's possible to enjoy without over-indulging. There are days too when I decide that it's a "Carb Day." For example, one very hot day in the summer warrants my once-a-year small ice cream or custard cone. Or if some kind person makes me a birthday cake I'll eat a bit. I call these excursions "experimental error." I am not perfect, but I try to keep my carbohydrate intake under 50 g/day and ideally around 30 g/day. For me, the lower my carbohydrate, the far better my control.

Wendy Knapp Pogozelski earned a BS from Chatham University and a PhD in chemistry from Johns Hopkins University under the direction of Thomas Tullius. She spent two years as an Office of Naval Research postdoctoral fellow working at various sites in radiation biology. She is a professor of chemistry at the State University of New York (SUNY) College at Geneseo, where she has been since 1996. She teaches biochemistry, emphasizing medical and nutrition-based applications. Her current research focuses on radiation effects on mitochondrial function and mitochondrial DNA as well as on understanding how dietary strategies affect biochemical pathways.

CHAPTER 11

Metabolic Syndrome

The Big Pitch

Through the last two chapters, we've learned that diabetes represents the most clear-cut example of how the glucose–insulin axis affects health. Diabetes rests at the center of nutritional thinking, whether or not you are a patient yourself. If you are primarily interested in weight loss or cardiovascular disease (CVD)—or even if your concern is general good health—insulin metabolism is always in the foreground. The focal point of so many of the issues we've discussed is metabolic syndrome (MetS). The idea is generally credited to Gerald Reaven, an endocrinologist who died in 2018 at age eighty-nine. His original observation, which sparked the idea of MetS, was that overweight, high blood glucose, high blood pressure, and the lipid markers assumed to indicate cardiovascular risk commonly appeared together in the same patients (table 11.1). [1] MetS is not a disease but rather a collection of physiological markers that represent risk of disease. The separate components of the syndrome are not just superficially related, either. Reaven's insight was to suggest that the markers arose from some common central cause, which he, and most of us, see as disruption in the glucose–insulin axis.

The concept has now been extended to include several other physiologic markers, including inflammation and LDL particle size, that also seem to be tied together. Insulin is credited with control of the syndrome, and fittingly, several years before his death, Reaven insisted that MetS should be called "insulin-resistance syndrome." [2]

The importance of metabolic syndrome came through to me a few years ago. I was listening to a presentation at a seminar on metabolic syndrome and its underlying cell biology. I don't remember the details of the presentation, but I thought it was quite good. The speaker was also a doctor—in

Table 11.1. National Cholesterol Education Program Adult Treatment Panel III Definition of Metabolic Syndrome—Subjects have three of the following criteria

	Men	Women
Abdominal obesity, waist circumference	> 40 inches	> 35 inches
Hypertriglyceridemia	> 150 mg/dL	> 150 mg/dL
Low HDL-cholesterol	< 40 mg/dL	< 50 mg/dL
High blood pressure	> 130/85 mm Hg	> 130/85 mm Hg
High fasting glucose	> 110 mg/dL	> 110 mg/dL

Source: NCEP Expert Panel on Detection, Evaluation, and Treatment of High Blood Cholesterol in Adults (Bethesda, MD: National Institutes of Health, 2001).

fact, he was Mike Huckabee's doctor. After the seminar, I asked him about low-carbohydrate diets and he unexpectedly went ballistic. "Go to the Atkins website. You can eat all the bacon you want. That's what it says." I was somewhat taken aback. Did I say Atkins? I didn't really know what to say. I noticed that he still had on the screen his last slide showing the criteria for metabolic syndrome (something like table 11.1).

Pointing to the screen, I said, "You know, all of those markers are exactly the things that are improved by low-carb diets." He said, "Well, they're also improved by low-calorie diets," which is simply not true. Low-fat diets, or at least high-carbohydrate diets, will not improve triglycerides and other markers, and will more likely make them worse. Plus the level of blood glucose is determined by carbohydrate in the diet. Everybody agrees on that.

The incident stuck in my head. A little later that day it occurred to me that I might have said something smart. The features of MetS were known to be improved by carbohydrate restriction, but this was not generally stated explicitly, or maybe its full import was not realized. Turning it around in your mind, you might say that the response to a low-carbohydrate diet could actually be the essential feature of metabolic syndrome, a kind of operational definition.

The existence of a syndrome—that is, the simultaneous appearance of the markers—is no longer in question. It is also widely accepted that the syndrome might be a reflection of insulin resistance. Yet the full impact of MetS has not yet been appreciated. Its clinical importance continues to be questioned by some critics who claim that MetS is not a useful idea. These critics hold that saying your patient has the markers of MetS provides no more information than the primary observation that the markers do in fact often show up together. What they mean is that, whatever the underlying causes, the only way to treat markers A, B, and C (for example, obesity, diabetes, and high cholesterol) is with a drug for A, a drug for B, and a drug for C. In other words, they don't have a single drug for MetS—only for each of the individual markers.

The fact that A, B, and C can all be treated with a single intervention, namely, a low-carbohydrate diet, suggests that all the markers do in fact arise from a common cause: a disruption in the glucose–insulin axis, roughly described as insulin resistance. Low-carbohydrate diets could thus provide a working definition of the syndrome. If your patient had the markers traditionally associated with MetS and they improved with a low-carbohydrate diet, it would confirm that the patient did indeed have metabolic syndrome. I knew this was a good idea because other people had brought it up before. I had even written a paper myself titled "Metabolic Syndrome and Low-Carbohydrate Ketogenic Diets in the Medical School Biochemistry Curriculum," but I hadn't really seen the impact. There is a step in the evolution of ideas when you realize that a comment you made in passing has important implications and has to be restated as a law.

If all the markers of metabolic syndrome could be improved by a low-carbohydrate diet, possibly even in the absence of calorie restriction, than what would that mean for the millions of people facing the risk predicted by these markers? What would it mean for the drugs that treat each individual condition but ignore the root cause? Lastly, what would it mean for those national authorities on health that were, and are still, recommending a low-fat, high-carbohydrate diet? If the experimental data are there, would the nutritional establishment embrace them, even though they contain the words "low-carbohydrate"? It was 2005 and we really thought that progress could be made. Talk about the naïveté of youth.

Jeff Volek and I went through the literature and tabulated the responses to low-carbohydrate and low-fat diets with respect to the markers of MetS. The results, which we published in *Nutrition and Metabolism*,[3] were as we expected (figure 11.1). I was the editor of *Nutrition and Metabolism* at the time and thought that the paper would improve the standing of our journal. We recognized that we were dealing with modern science, where people don't even have time to read an abstract, so we put the whole story in the title: "Carbohydrate Restriction Improves the Features of Metabolic Syndrome. Metabolic Syndrome May Be Defined by the Response to Carbohydrate Restriction." The data showed that except for a couple of measurements (insulin, fasting glucose), the markers of MetS are improved by a low-carbohydrate diet, sometimes dramatically. Probably the best indicator of CVD risk based on commonly measured parameters is the ratio of triglycerides:HDL where the reduction is typically three to ten times greater in carbohydrate reduction.

Volek's Test of the Theory

In chapter 7, we looked at the experiments in Jeff Volek's laboratory showing that saturated fat in the blood was reduced by a low-carbohydrate diet with high saturated fat, as compared to low-fat diet with low saturated fat. The results on control of plasma saturated fat are critical because the presence of dietary saturated fat is still held up as an objection against low-carbohydrate diets. It was also the magnitude of the effect in Volek's experiment that was surprising. The total SFA fraction in the low-carbohydrate group was reduced by more than half, and this reduction was more than three times the average change in the low-fat group.

This study had a larger overall significance, however. The real power of Volek's experiments was that the participants all fit the definition of metabolic syndrome, and that a wide variety of lipid and physiologic parameters were measured. Figure 11.1 shows that everything got better: HDL, insulin, leptin, and most dramatically, triglycerides.

The Pitch

This chapter reinforces the big pitch: If the coincidence of metabolic markers that defines MetS indicates a unified mechanism, if seemingly different physiologic effects—overweight, high blood pressure, atherogenic dyslipidemia, high triglycerides, low HDL, high blood glucose, high insulin—are all a reflection of a common underlying stimulus (proposed to

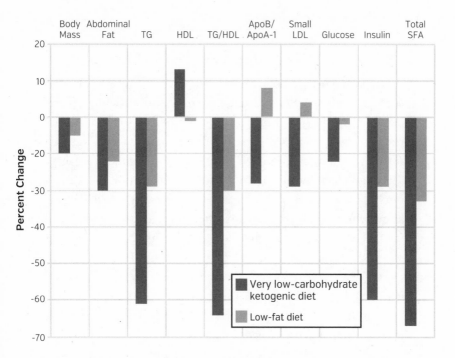

Figure 11.1. Summary of responses of forty people with metabolic syndrome to a very low-carbohydrate ketogenic diet (VLCKD) or a low-fat diet (LFD). Data from J. S. Volek et al., "Carbohydrate Restriction Has a More Favorable Impact on the Metabolic Syndrome than a Low Fat Diet," *Lipids* 44, no. 4 (2009): 297–309.

be disruption in insulin metabolism), then if we can treat any one of those features, we can treat them all.

Nothing is better than low-carbohydrate for weight loss, but other diets do work. It's harder for women and it's harder as you get older, but there are lots of ways to get thinner. We don't really have the answer on CVD. We know a lot of things that might be relevant but we don't really know the fundamental cause. However, what we do know with some certainty is about diabetes: Cutting back on carbohydrate is the most effective treatment. For many it is a virtual cure. In the long term, it is better than drugs. So if MetS is really a clue to an underlying mechanism for all of the disparate markers, then effectively treating hyperglycemia will improve all of the features of MetS—that is to say, we have a prescription for general health.

The Head-and-Shoulders Effect

In addition to metabolic effects, a low-carbohydrate diet will cure irritable bowel syndrome and related disorders in many people. (Cancer is waiting in the wings, too.) In some sense, the problem with convincing people of the benefits of a reduced carbohydrate strategy is that it appears to be good for everything, good for what ails you. You can sound like a hard-sell pitchman. I call this the Head-and-Shoulders effect. I don't know whether it is true but a rep from Procter & Gamble once told me that when they first brought out the shampoo of that name, they advertised that it would cure your dandruff in three days. What their tests actually showed was that it would cure it in one day, but they didn't think anybody would believe that. It is probably not that low-carbohydrate is so good but that high-carbohydrate is so bad.

PART 4

The Mess in Nutritional Science

CHAPTER 12

The Medical Literature
A Guide to Flawed Studies

Nutrition is in crisis. Almost every day a new study shows that you are at risk for diabetes, cardiovascular disease, or all-cause mortality brought on by a newly identified toxin that turns out to be something that you just had for lunch. It is not clear that any of these studies are subject to serious critical peer review, and for the curious, bloggers usually do a good job of dismembering them. The continuous cycle of weak studies and their deconstruction goes beyond mere time wasting. People are hurt because bad recommendations are left out there, even when research shows that they are inappropriate—and, in the process, science takes a big hit. The editors and reviewers of technical and medical journals who conduct peer review are supposed to act as the gatekeepers of scientific evidence, but the journals continue to publish papers showing very weak associations, and even some that are grossly misleading or contradictory. The media, which might be expected to help our case, make it worse. It's not really their fault. A science reporter cannot reasonably have the time to read the original study in detail, and must instead accept the conclusions in the abstract, and so that message is transmitted through mass media. When you do explain to the reporter how misleading these reports are, and how people will be hurt, they are truly concerned and sympathetic, but they don't always have complete editorial control. In any case they would like to help, but tomorrow they have to cover a story that may be even worse. It is really hard for the consumer. This post from Facebook probably tells the story: "So epically confused about diet. Everything I read is contradictory on epic proportions. About the only consistencies are low-sugar raw veggies and water. How in the world is a girl to sort it out, other than try everything and see what works for me?"

She went on to ask why it isn't "possible to come up with a system that takes inputs—body stats and genetic history—and outputs a general reasonable diet to follow?" Chances are that the population at large is no more comfortable than this woman on Facebook when it comes to matters of nutrition. I wrote to her through private messages and reiterated the first three rules: (1) If you are okay, you are okay; (2) if you want to lose weight, don't eat, and if you have to eat, don't eat carbs; and (3) if you have diabetes or metabolic syndrome, you have to try a low-carbohydrate diet first.

It is likely that many people wind up believing nothing at all, however, and simply assume that everything is exaggerated, save for the most ingrained popular notion that "maybe fat is bad and maybe I should not put so much salt on my food." Then there is the progression of articles on raspberry-ketones, resveratrol, trans-fats, and methylglyoxal, each of which will either kill you or save you, depending on whom you ask.

Most discouraging are the health agencies. The American Diabetes Association (ADA) wants people with diabetes to consume a lot of carbo- hydrates. They keep saying that they don't have a diet, and that they're not opposed to low-carbohydrate diets (for weight loss)—but instead they stress "individualization" without any indication as to which individuals benefit from which intervention. Despite the disclaimers and ever-shifting language, there is no doubt that the ADA is perceived as opposing low- carbohydrate—and it seems clear they are the only ones responsible for that perception.

The evidence that weight loss is not required for improvement in diabe- tes, from the work of Nuttall and Gannon,[1] for example, is not mentioned by the ADA. They know about that evidence. I'm sure of it because I have told members of the committee personally, and they should already be aware because some of the work was funded by the ADA itself. The ADA guidelines do not cite important scientific work showing that weight loss is not required for improvement in diabetes. People who are not scientists ask me, understandably incredulous, "Can you do that? Are you allowed to make recommendations without citing other people's work?"

There is a daily progression of sweeping statements that go way beyond the published data. At the same time there remains an inability or an unwill- ingness to zero in on real factors. The low-carbohydrate diet has attained the status of the name of God in Hebrew: It must never be said out loud.

Part of the problem is that the literature, especially major medical publications, is still predominantly subscription-based. Most people cannot access the information, so the results are then fed downstream to the media, who take anything they are fed at face value, and then pass it on further to the general public.

The rigid dogma of the literature has reached Galilean proportions. Fructose and sugar are bad (unless you try to lump them in with all carbohydrates). If you want your paper on fructose to be published, begin with: "Because of the deleterious effects of dietary fructose, we hypothesized that . . ." Never start with: "Whether dietary fructose has a deleterious effect . . ." Our paper on fructose was published with "whether . . ." as the opening sentence,[2] but only after a hard-fought rebuttal of reviewers' criticisms that turned out to be fifteen pages long. Worse, if you even mention low-carbohydrate, you are guaranteed real grief. When the *Journal of the American Medical Association* published George Bray's "calorie-is-a-calorie"[3] and I pointed out that the study more accurately supported the importance of carbohydrate as a controlling variable, the editor refused to publish my letter. Thankfully, blogs have performed a valuable service by providing an alternative point of view, but if unreliability is a problem in the scientific literature, that problem is multiplied exponentially in internet sources. In the end, consumers might feel that they are pretty much on their own.

It does take some confidence, especially for the layperson, to feel that their intuitive understanding is correct: that the difference between white rice and brown rice is so small that it really doesn't matter what Harvard's computer says. Most researchers are very much disinclined to get into a shooting match, or worse, whistle-blowing. The long blue line is a strong force in repressing investigation, not because the authorities think corruption is okay, but because scandal reflects badly on everybody. Whistle-blowing in this field is especially weird because sometimes the transgressions are right out in the open.

Statistics: Death of the Medical Literature

Many scientists believe that if you do a good experiment, you don't need statistics. David Colquohon, a well-known neuroscientist and critic of

The Golden Rule of Statistics

Here's the Golden Rule for reading a scientific paper, from the book *PDQ Statistics* by Norman and Streiner: "The important point . . . is that the onus is on the author to convey to the reader an accurate impression of what the data look like, using graphs or standard measures, before beginning the statistical shenanigans. Any paper that doesn't do this should be viewed from the outset with considerable suspicion."[4]

In other words, explain things clearly to the reader. There are complicated ideas in science but the often quoted statement (only once before in this book) from Einstein, that you should make it simple but not too simple, is a reasonable demand for you, the reader, to make of the scientific literature.

poor scientific method, agrees. Colquohon is the author of an excellent, if technical, statistics book, which is now freely available online.[5] The introduction to his book points out: "The snag, of course, is that doing good experiments is difficult. Most people need all the help they can get to prevent them making fools of themselves by claiming that their favorite theory is substantiated by observations that do nothing of the sort."

This kind of circumspection is, unfortunately, more common among people who write the statistics books than those who use them. A good statistics book will have an introduction that says something like "In statistics, we try to put a number on our intuition." In other words, it is not really, by itself, a science. It is, or should be, a tool for the experimenter's use, and like any tool, you have to know how to use it. Because statistics offers so many tools, there is not always agreement on which hammer goes with which nail. All of statistics is interpretation. The problem is that many authors of papers in the medical literature allow statistics to become their master rather than their servant: Numbers are plugged into a statistical program and the results are interpreted in a cut-and-dried fashion. Statistical significance (that two sets of data are not from the same population) is confused with clinical significance (that differences are sufficiently large to have a biological effect). Misuse of statistics is the subject of numerous papers and books, but this has had little effect.

Statistical Shenanigans versus Common Sense

How do you deal with the reports in the press that tell you that white rice will give you diabetes but brown rice won't? The saving principle is that, despite its subtleties and reliance on mathematics, biochemistry uses the same basic rules of logic as daily life. So the first question you have to ask is whether a given study makes sense: How is it possible that white rice is so different from brown rice? A moment's thought suggests that the major difference between the two is in the stuff that isn't even digested, the fiber. The nutritional establishment is always pushing fiber—whole grain and all that—so you might want to hear their case, but then there is the possibility that the entire fiber thing itself is questionable or at least exaggerated—and what of the Asian societies that are always invoked to tell us how much we need grain, yet never ate brown rice. Never. So, it can be confusing, and common sense makes you suspicious.

Habeas Corpus Datorum

Science is an extension of common sense, but that doesn't mean there aren't revolutionary ideas. You want to be suspicious of a revolutionary idea if it violates common sense, but you can't throw out the idea just for that reason. The solution is simple, if not always easy to implement: If it is a reasonable conclusion, you can cut the author some slack. If the idea is far out, you need to see the data—all the data—not just the average of the data or conclusions from the computer. My new grand principle of doing science: *habeas corpus datorum*. Let's see the body of the data. If the conclusion is nonintuitive and goes against previous work or common sense, then the data must be strong and clearly presented.

So, how should you read a scientific paper? I usually want to see the pictures, or figures, first. It's not just about saving a thousand words, as the saying goes. It's about presentation of the data, and it's about the Golden Rule of Statistics: "Convey to the reader an accurate impression of what the data look like, using graphs or standard measures, before beginning the statistical shenanigans." On the topic of tables: Figures are so much better than tables that a whole book, *Medical Illuminations*, was written about the idea.[6]

Many of us write scientific papers in the same way we read them. We make the figures first and then try to figure out what they say. The principle: A scientific paper is supposed to explain. I tell graduate students that if you do an experiment and you don't explain it well, it's as if you never did it at all. In teaching students how to present their work, I ask them: "Describe what you are supposed to do in a scientific seminar or other presentation." Sometimes they begin to say something, but I usually make it worse by adding: "No. In one word. What are you supposed to do? One word." Having reached an appropriate level of annoyance where they will be relieved to hear the answer, I give it to them: "Teach." You want to explain things to your audience. The same is true of a scientific paper. Again, the Golden Rule of Statistics: The onus is on the author.

Caveat Lector

Presenting a scientific paper is also a bit like selling something. Scientific papers are rarely just data. They have an idea that they are trying to sell. Teaching and selling are the two things you do in science. The reader has to be an educated consumer, however, and as an educated consumer she or he should be suspicious of overselling. One good indicator of overselling is the use of value judgments as if they were scientific terms. "Healthy" (or "healthful") is not a scientific term.

If a study describes a diet as "healthy," it is almost guaranteed to be a flawed study. If we knew which diets were "healthy," we wouldn't have an obesity epidemic. A good example is the paper by Appel on the DASH diet, which concluded: "In the setting of a healthful diet, partial substitution of carbohydrate with either protein or monounsaturated fat can further lower blood pressure, improve lipid levels, and reduce estimated cardiovascular risk."[7]

It's hard to know how healthful the original diet could have been if removing carbohydrate improved everything. In addition, not only was this about a "carbohydrate-rich diet used in the DASH trials" but it is "currently advocated in several scientific reports." Another red flag is when the authors tell you how widely accepted their idea is.

Understatement is good. One of the more famous is from the classic Watson and Crick paper of 1953, in which the two researchers proposed the DNA double helix structure. They said, "It has not escaped our notice that the specific pairing we have postulated immediately suggests a possible copying mechanism for the genetic material."

What Is Wrong with the Literature and What Is Right

Let's start with what's right. There are many published papers in the nutritional literature that are informative, creative, and generally conform to the standards of good science. Naturally, like any scientific literature, most papers are fairly routine. They are of specialized interest, or—as described in one of the choices on the checklist for referees who review manuscripts—"of interest to other workers in the field."

What's wrong is not the mediocre papers but rather the surprising number of really objectionable papers. The medical literature is full of papers bordering on fraud, or at least, guilty of misrepresentation. There are many papers that are full of fundamental errors and total lack of judgment in interpretation. Worse, there is a possibility that somebody is going to get hurt because of bad medical advice that follows from these misinterpretations.

Most work in most fields, more or less by definition, is mediocre. What makes papers in medical nutrition different is their drastic claims about saving hundreds of thousands of lives by scaling up a result that had hardly any effect to begin with to the entire population.

It is difficult to face the fact that so much of the medical literature is published by people who are not trained in science, which means they don't know the game, they haven't seen much of it, and they wouldn't know good science if they saw it. There is no real conceptual training in science. You can learn techniques, but it's not about cyclotrons, it's about ideas. There is no reason why a physician can't do real scientific thinking, but at the same time, there is no reason why he or she can. An MD degree is not a guarantee of any expertise outside the practitioner's area of specialty.

The irony is that the practice of medicine can be highly scientific. Differential diagnosis and the experience in recommending the right drug are the kinds of things that are part of scientific disciplines. The same physician who will intuitively solve a medical mystery, though, will assume that, for scientific research, things are different—that there are somehow arbitrary rules and that brute-force application of statistics will tell you whether what you did is true.

The next six chapters will detail the failures of nutritional literature, ranging from the slightly inaccurate—"association does not imply causality" (sometimes it does and sometimes it doesn't)—to the idiotic—"you must do intention-to-treat" (if you assign subjects to take a drug and they don't take it, you have to include their data with those who did). I will also cover "levels of evidence": arbitrary rules that get incorporated into tables, the top of which is always some kind of "gold standard." The odd thing about levels of scientific evidence is that nobody in any physical science would recognize them. They are, in fact, the creation of people who are trying to do science but wouldn't know science if they saw it—fundamentally amateurs who have arbitrary rules along the lines of the apocryphal story about Mozart:

> A man comes to Mozart and wants to become a composer. Mozart says that he has to study theory for a couple of years, that he should study orchestration and become proficient at the piano, and goes on like this. Finally the man says, "But you wrote your first symphony when you were eight years old." Mozart says, "Yes, but I didn't ask anybody."

The Bottom Line

To understand research in nutrition, or really, any science, one has to be prepared to question "the experts." If a paper does not adhere to the Golden Rule and is too quick to begin "the statistical shenanigans," it "should be viewed from the outset with considerable suspicion."

The bottom line is that you have to expect real communication from the authors of a scientific paper. The problem, for many people, lies in the difficulty of believing that the best and the brightest are at fault. But it is not hard to find examples of experts making mistakes. I will try to provide you with all the help I can in the following chapters.

CHAPTER 13

Observational Studies, Association, Causality

789 deaths were reported in Doll and Hill's original cohort. Thirty-six of these were attributed to lung cancer. When these lung cancer deaths were counted in smokers versus non-smokers, the correlation virtually sprang out: all thirty-six of the deaths had occurred in smokers. The difference between the two groups was so significant that Doll and Hill did not even need to apply complex statistical metrics to discern it. The trial designed to bring the most rigorous statistical analysis to the cause of lung cancer barely required elementary mathematics to prove his point.

—Siddhartha Mukherjee,
The Emperor of All Maladies

Scientists don't like philosophy of science. It is not just that pompous phrases like *hypothetico-deductive systems* are such a turnoff; it's that we rarely recognize descriptions of science in philosophy articles as accurate reflections of what we actually do. In the end, there is no definition of science any more than there is a definition for music or for literature. Because scientists have different styles, it is hard to generalize about actual scientific behavior. Research is a human activity, and precisely because it puts a premium on creativity, it defies categorization. As the physicist Steven Weinberg put it, echoing Justice Stewart on pornography: "There is no logical formula that establishes a sharp dividing line between a beautiful explanatory theory and a mere list of data, but we know the difference when we see it—we demand a simplicity and rigidity in our principles before we are willing to take them seriously."[1]

We know, however, that what we see in the current state of nutrition is not "a beautiful explanatory theory" or anything of the sort. This forces us to consider what it is that makes nutritional medical literature so bad. If we can identify some principles, maybe we can penetrate the mess and see how it could be fixed.

One frequently stated principle is that "observational studies only generate hypotheses." There is the related principle that "association does not imply causality," usually cited in a backhanded way by those authors who want you to believe that the association they found does in fact imply causality. These two principles are not exactly right. They fail to recognize that scientific experiments are not so easily wedged into categories like "observational studies." Principles like "observational studies only generate hypotheses" are also widely invoked by bloggers and critics to discredit the continuing stream of observational studies that make an association between their favored targets—eggs, red meat, sugar-sweetened soda—and prevalence of some metabolic disease or cancer. In most cases, the original studies are getting what they deserve, but the bills of indictment are not accurate, and it would be better not to cite absolute statements of scientific principles. It is not simply that these studies are observational studies, but rather that they are bad observational studies, and in many cases, the associations that they find are so weak that the study—if anything—constitutes an argument against causality. On the assumption that good experimental practice and interpretation could be roughly defined, I laid out a few principles that I thought were a better representation—if you can even make such generalization—of what actually goes on in science:

- Observations generate hypotheses. Observational studies test hypotheses. Associations do not necessarily imply causality. In some sense, all science is associations.
- Only mathematics is axiomatic (starts from absolute assumptions).
- If you notice that kids who eat a lot of candy seem to be fat, or even if you notice that you yourself get fat eating candy, that is an observation. From this observation, you might come up with the hypothesis that sugar causes obesity. Thus, an observation generates hypotheses. A test of your hypothesis would be to carry out an observational study. For example, you might try to see if there is an association between sugar consumption and

incidence of obesity. There are different ways of doing this—the simplest epidemiologic approach is simply to compare the history of the eating behavior of individuals (insofar as you can get it) with how fat they are. When you do this comparison you are testing your hypothesis.

For the final point on the list, you must remember that there are an infinite number of other things—meat consumption, TV hours, distance from a French bakery, grandfather's waist circumference—that you could have measured as an independent variable. Your hypothesis, however, is that the variable is candy. What about all the others? Mike Eades, author of the influential *Protein Power*, described falling asleep as a child by trying to think of everything in the world. You just can't test them all. As Einstein put it, "Your theory determines the measurement you make." If you found associations with everything, would anything be causal?

Association Can Predict Causality

In fact, association can provide strong evidence for causation. If we didn't ask about the extent to which the tacos we ate were the cause of our stomach upset, we would not function well in our daily lives. Single observations might generate a hypothesis or a guess that we can test. We can determine, for example, whether a particular restaurant is good through continuous "testing." Single observations generate hypotheses. Hypotheses, in turn, generate observational studies, not the other way around. A correct statement is that association does not *necessarily* imply causation. In some sense, all science is observation and association. Even thermodynamics, the most mathematical and absolute of sciences, rests on observation. We have never observed a true perpetual motion machine, so we have generalized that observation into a physical law, but as soon as somebody makes one that works, it's all over.

Biological mechanisms, or perhaps all scientific theories, are never proved. By legal analogy: You cannot be found innocent, only not guilty. That is why excluding a theory is stronger than showing consistency. The grand epidemiological study of macronutrient intake—the association of what Americans ate in the last forty years and the incidence of diabetes and obesity—shows that increased carbohydrate is associated with increased calories, even under conditions where fruits and vegetables also go up and where fat, if anything, goes down. The data on dietary consumption and disease in the whole population can be described as an observational study, but it is strong because it gives support to a lack of causal effect of decreased fat on positive outcome—it excludes a theory.

Again, in science, finding a contradiction has greater impact than merely finding a consistent result. The multitude of prospective experiments (where you pick the population first and see how people do on your variable of interest) have shown in the past, and will undoubtedly continue to show, the same lack of relation between fat intake and disease. But will anybody give up on saturated fat? In a court of law, if you are found not guilty of child abuse, people may still not let you move into their neighborhood. An association will tell you about causality if: (1) the association is strong; (2) there is a plausible underlying mechanism; and (3) there is not a more plausible explanation.

The often-cited coincidental correlation between cardiovascular disease and number of TV sets does not imply causality because, although the first principle of observational studies is observed, there is no logical direct underlying mechanism. TV does not cause CVD. Interestingly, in the case of CVD, where so many associations have been published, and so many learned societies have told us how to prevent or cure the disease, there remains little in the way of an agreed upon mechanism.

Re-Inventing the Wheel: Me and Bradford Hill

This chapter is a reworking of a blog post that I published in 2013. The post included the principles I laid out at the top of the chapter for dealing with the kind of observational studies that you see in the scientific literature. I was speaking off the top of my head, trying to describe the logic that scientists use in interpreting data. It was an obvious description of what is done in practice. I didn't think it was particularly original, and again, I don't think that there are any hard and fast principles in science. When I described what I had written to my colleague, Dr. Eugene Fine, his response was, "Aren't you re-inventing the wheel?" He meant that Bradford Hill, pretty much the inventor of modern epidemiology, had already established these and a couple of others as principles. In our conversation, Eugene cited *The Emperor of All Maladies*,[2] an outstanding book on the history of cancer. I had, in fact, read *Emperor* on his recommendation. I remembered Bradford Hill and the description of the evolution of the ideas of epidemiology, population studies, and randomized controlled trials. The story is also told in James LeFanu's *The Rise and Fall of Modern Medicine*,[3] another captivating history of medicine.

I thought of these as general philosophical ideas, rather than as absolute scientific principles. Perhaps it is that we're just used to it, but saying that an association has to be very strong to imply causality is common sense, and not in the same ballpark with the Pythagorean theorem. It's something that you might say over coffee or in response to somebody's blog. Being explicit about it turns out to be very important, but like much in philosophy of science, it struck me as not of great intellectual import. It all reminded me of learning, in grade school, that the Earl of Sandwich had invented the sandwich. At which time I thought, "This is an invention?" Woody Allen thought the same thing years later and wrote the history of the sandwich. He recorded the Earl's early failures: "In 1741, he places bread on bread with turkey on top. This fails. In 1745, he exhibits bread with turkey on either side. Everyone rejects this except David Hume."

In fact, Hill's principles remain important even if seemingly obvious. The pervasive violation of these principles in the medical literature constitutes their real significance. The concept of the randomized controlled trial (RCT)—randomly assigning people to a drug or behavior that you're testing, or to a group that is the control—while obvious to us now, was hard won. Likewise, proving that any particular environmental factor—diet, smoking, pollution, or toxic chemicals—was the cause of a disease, and that by reducing that factor, the disease could be prevented, turned out to be a very hard sell, especially to physicians whose view of disease might have been strongly colored by the idea of an infective agent, bacterium, or virus.

The Rise and Fall of Modern Medicine describes Bradford Hill's two important contributions[4]: He demonstrated that tuberculosis could be cured by a combination of two drugs, streptomycin and PAS (para-aminosalicylic acid), and even more importantly, he showed that tobacco causes lung cancer. Hill was a professor of medical statistics at the London School of Hygiene and Tropical Medicine, but was not formally trained in statistics, and like many of us, thought of proper statistics simply as applied common sense. Ironically, an early near-fatal case of tuberculosis prevented formal medical education. His first monumental accomplishment was, in fact, to demonstrate how tuberculosis was cured by the streptomycin–PAS combination. In 1941, Hill and his coworker Richard Doll undertook a systematic investigation of the risk factors for lung cancer. His eventual success was accompanied by a description of the principles that allow you to say when association can be taken as causation.

Association and Causality: The Nine Criteria

Bradford Hill described the factors that might lead you to believe that an association supports a causal role. Hill's criteria are still perfectly reasonable today, though in the current medical literature, they are probably much more widely practiced in the breach than the observance. The diligent application of Hill's principles to the medical literature would substantially reduce the size of the literature and improve the quality of what remained:

1. STRENGTH. "First upon my list I would put the strength of the association," Hill wrote. This, of course, is exactly what is missing in the continued epidemiological scare stories whose measures of relative risk are so small. Hill describes:

> Prospective inquiries into smoking have shown that the death rate from cancer of the lung in cigarette smokers is nine to ten times the rate in non-smokers and the rate in heavy cigarette smokers is twenty to thirty times as great. . . . On the other hand the death rate from coronary thrombosis in smokers is no more than twice, possibly less, than the death rate in non-smokers. Though there is good evidence to support causation it is surely much easier in this case to think of some features of life that may go hand-in-hand with smoking—features that might conceivably be the real underlying cause or, at the least, an important contributor, whether it be lack of exercise, nature of diet or other factors.

Hill expressed doubts about a relative risk of 2 or less. Criticized elsewhere in this book, relative risk (RR) is what it sounds like: the ratio of the risks from two outcomes. Risk is the probability of an outcome; relative risk is the ratio of the individual risks of two events. For example, if you were to compare a group of factory workers in a chemical plant, say, to the general population and you found that for every 1,000 workers, 26 developed cancer, then the probability, the risk of cancer is 26 out of 1,000 or 0.026 or 2.6 percent. If you found in the general population that there were only 13 cases of cancer for every 1,000 people, then the risk for the general population is 13 out of 1,000 or 0.013 or 1.3 percent. You can then calculate relative risk as follows:

$$RR = (\text{risk for workers}) / (\text{risk for population}) = (26/1,000) / (13/1,000) = 2{:}1$$

This might be considered evidence for environmental hazard, although as Hill says, it would be stronger if the RR were 10. Still 2 is considered grounds for taking the results seriously (or taking the factory owner to court). RR, however, as its name suggests, is relative. It hides information. The RR would still be 2 if there were 26 out of a million workers getting sick and 13 out of a million in the general population. The absolute risk is the difference between the probabilities. Absolute risk in this example is small (2.6 percent–1.3 percent = 1.3 percent). In other words, not even a full 2 percent more factory workers got cancer than the general population. If you did take the factory owner to court, the judge might ask for additional evidence.

This is what are we up against. Even within the limitations of relative risk, the way in which the results are presented can significantly affect a reader's perception. The abstract from a study on eating breakfast found that: "Men who skipped breakfast had a 27% higher risk of CHD compared with men who did not."[5] The number 27 percent sounds a great deal more impressive than the relative risk of 1.27, even though the latter might paint a better picture of the limited effects. For every 227 people with cancer, 100 will be regular breakfast eaters and 127 will have passed. By Hill's standards, or by common sense, a relative risk of 1.27 would not make you force yourself to eat breakfast if you weren't hungry. Describing the results as "27% higher risk," on the other hand, might influence your behavior more. Reporting relative risk so as to make the effect larger is the single most prevalent mistake in the medical literature and is even worse in the media that report on that literature. It must be noted, however, that while a high relative risk is no guarantee of causality, a low relative risk is definitely suspicious.

2. CONSISTENCY. Hill listed the repetition of the results of studies, under different circumstances, as a criterion for considering the extent to which an association implied causality. We expect results to be reproducible, and a weak association might gain some strength if the observation is reproduced. Consistency of strong results, however, is what we want to see.

Criterion 2 is not, however, independent of criterion 1. Although Hill himself did not mention this, it is of great importance. Consistently weak associations do not generally add up to a strong association. If there is a single practice in modern medicine that is completely out of whack with respect to careful consideration of causality, it is the use of meta-analyses where studies with marginal strengths are averaged to create a conclusion that is stronger than the majority of its components. In fact, many meta-analyses include studies that have not shown any association at all; the authors average them with a couple that have and then report the average as significant. Averaging studies without significant outcomes and expecting to get an effect is as foolish as it sounds, but it is widely practiced.

3. SPECIFICITY. Hill was circumspect on this point, recognizing that we should have an open mind on what causes what. On specificity in the study of cancer and cigarettes, Hill noted that the two sites where he had showed a cause-and-effect relationship were the lungs and the nose.

4. TEMPORALITY. Obviously we expect the cause to precede the effect. Hill recognized that temporality was not so clear for diseases that developed slowly. "Does a particular diet lead to disease or do the early stages of the disease lead to those peculiar dietetic habits?" Of current interest are the epidemiologic studies that show a correlation between diet soda and obesity. These studies are quick to assert a causal link, but there is always a question of which way causation proceeds. One might reasonably ask, "What kind of people drink diet sodas?" The kind of people who want to lose weight. Most important from the temporal perspective, carbohydrate restriction has immediate and dramatic effects on a disease, diabetes, that has severe acute symptoms. The fact that the "concerns" about long-term effects have never actually materialized pretty much defines the crisis in nutrition.

5. BIOLOGICAL GRADIENT. Association should show a dose–response curve. In the case of cigarettes, the death rate from cancer of the lung increases linearly with the number of cigarettes smoked. A subset of the first principle—that the association should be strong—is that the dose–response curve should have a meaningful slope—that is, the difference between the numbers at the beginning and the end of the scale should be substantial, and of course, should not show large fluctuations. Numerous studies in the literature can avoid putting their results to the test by lumping data into quartile. When fifty points are lumped into one quartile, it might show slope, but it would be nice to know the gradient within each quartile.

6. PLAUSIBILITY. Hill said, "What is biologically plausible depends upon the biological knowledge of the day." Here, Hill's emphasis on effect size is important. If the association is far-fetched, unexpected, or derived from a less-than-obvious idea, there is a greater burden of proof and any association should be strong.

7. COHERENCE. Data, according to Hill, "should not seriously conflict with the generally known facts of the natural history and biology of the disease." The natural history of diabetes is the effect of carbohydrate—not fat, not red meat, not any protein. Any number of other factors might be involved, but if you don't put carbohydrate first, you are giving up on the common sense that Hill acknowledged was the basis of his criteria.

8. EXPERIMENT. It was another age. It is hard to believe that it was in my lifetime that Hill proposed this principle: "Occasionally it is possible to appeal to experimental, or semi-experimental, evidence. For example, because of an observed association some preventive action is taken, does it, in fact, prevent?" The inventor of the randomized controlled trial would be amazed how many try to take preventative action, and how many, in fact, don't prevent—and most of all, he would have been astounded that it doesn't seem to affect the opinion of the medical community. The progression of failures, from the Framingham Study to the Women's Health Initiative, and the lack of association among low-fat, low saturated fat, and CVD, is strong evidence for the absence of causation.

9. ANALOGY. "In some circumstances it would be fair to judge by analogy. With the effects of thalidomide and rubella before us, we would surely be ready to accept slighter but similar evidence with another drug or another viral disease in pregnancy."

With the list concluded, this is Hill's final word on the criteria for determining causation:

Here then are nine different viewpoints from all of which we should study association before we cry causation. What I do not believe—and this has been suggested—is that we can usefully lay down some hard-and-fast rules of evidence that must be obeyed before we accept cause and effect. *None of my nine viewpoints can bring indisputable evidence for or against the cause-and-effect hypothesis and none can be required as a sine qua non.* What they can do, with greater or less strength, is to help us to make up our minds on the fundamental question—*is there any other way of explaining the set of facts before us, is there any other answer equally, or more, likely than cause and effect?* (Emphasis added)

This might be the first critique of the still-to-be-invented evidence-based medicine.

Nutritional Epidemiology

There are many critics of current nutritional epidemiology and most of us don't understand how the field could persist with so many weak results. It is simply the low standards and the failure to understand that statistics is not data, and it is not a science as such. Statistics comes from a particular person's opinion on how the data should be interpreted. Conflicts then arise from differing opinions. You must adjudicate between two principles: one, "The risk is small but when you scale it up to the whole population, you will save thousands of lives"; and two, to which I am partial, "When risk is small, there is low predictability of outcome. You can't scale up bad data."

The real impact of Hill's criteria is that they provide standards for interpreting epidemiological studies. They are standards that still have a good deal of subjectivity, but they are standards nonetheless. Yet they are ignored in nutrition. They are ignored by authors, and most importantly, they are ignored by the reviewers and editors who are expected to be the gatekeepers on solid science. In the end, the decision that an observational study implies causation is another way of saying that it is meaningful—that it is not an outcome of mathematical juggling—that it is, you know, science. *The Emperor of All Maladies* describes Hill's criteria as principles "which have remained in use by epidemiologists to date." But have they?

Many have voiced criticisms of epidemiology as it's currently practiced in nutrition. One way to look at the current problems in nutrition is that we have a large number of research groups doing epidemiology in violation of Hill's criteria.

Is It Science?

Science is a human activity. What we don't like about philosophy of science is that it is about the structure of science, rather than about what scientists really do, and so there aren't even any real definitions. Izja Lederhandler, a colleague at the NIH, put it well: "What you do in science is, you make a hypothesis and then you try to shoot yourself down." A good experiment puts the experimenter's theory to the test. An experiment whose outcome only shows consistency is not strong.

One of the most interesting insights on the work of Hill and Doll, as described in *The Emperor of All Maladies*, was that during breaks from the taxing work of analyzing the questionnaires on smoking, Doll himself would step out for a smoke. Doll believed that cigarettes were unlikely to be a cause—he favored tar from paved highways as the causative agent— but as the data came in, "in the middle of the survey, sufficiently alarmed, he gave up smoking."[6] In science, you try to shoot yourself down and you go with the data. The mass of papers demonizing fat, and the current flood of papers demonizing sugar, fail most of Hill's criteria. A major reason that they fail is that they set out to show consistency between the data and the theory, rather than to challenge the theory. They don't try to shoot themselves down. As a result, they don't consider what other facts could equally explain the data.

Navigating the Mess

The goal of this chapter, and those that surround it, is to help the consumer— and perhaps other scientists—read scientific publications. There really are no set principles of science. The existence of a "gold standard"—that is, the one best type of experiment that answers all questions—is not recognized in any science. The best experiment is the one that answers the question at hand. Observational studies are appropriate if researchers can't intervene for practical or ethical reasons. Such experiments imply causality if they show strong associations and if they have underlying mechanisms in basic chemistry or biology.

Bradford Hill laid down principles for dealing with observational studies, which he recognized as attempts to turn common sense into practice. Hill's criteria, once again, are as follows:

1. Strength   4. Temporality   7. Coherence
2. Consistency   5. Biological gradient   8. Experiment
3. Specificity   6. Plausibility   9. Analogy

Hill showed a causal link between cigarettes and cancer because he found that deaths from lung cancer for cigarette smokers were nine to ten times that of nonsmokers, a ratio that went up to twenty for heavy smokers compared to nonsmokers. He was less sure about coronary thrombosis because the relative risk (RR) was in the range of 2:1. This standard is not even proposed in modern nutritional experimentation. A nearly continuous flow of papers in the medical literature showing that something that you eat will cause some disease you don't want to have, even if the RR is as low as 1.3, has marred the field substantially. The majority of epidemiologic studies, in fact, violate Hill's criteria.

The most important feature of scientific behavior is, again, the mind-set. You have to have the courage to try to shoot your own theory down. This is consistent with the general principle that excluding a hypothesis is always stronger than showing consistency. The problem in nutrition is that experimenters are trying to prove things, instead of trying to *dis*prove things.

CHAPTER 14

Red Meat and
the New Puritans

*Dost thou think, because thou art virtuous, there shall be no
more cakes and ale?*

—WILLIAM SHAKESPEARE, *Twelfth Night*

Experts on nutrition are like experts on sexuality. No matter how
professional they might be, in some way, they are always trying to
justify their own lifestyle. Sure that others should follow their own
standards of behavior, they are always tempted to save us from our own sins,
whether sexual or dietary. While our own New England Puritans were not
actually down on sex (as described in Sara Vowell's *Wordy Shipmates*, they
actually thought sex was an argument for God's existence), they did have
the obsessive and literal insistence on what God really wanted. Sin was on
their minds.

The new Puritans of contemporary America want to save us from red
meat. It is unknown whether Michael Pollan's *In Defense of Food*[1] was
reporting the news or making it, but Pollan's recommendation to limit
meat consumption has become commonplace. *Vegetarian Times* says that
3.2 percent of the US population is vegetarian, and the Harvard School of
Public Health thinks that they are the righteous few among us.

There are good reasons for avoiding meat—better not to kill
anything, generally—but for most people, the health angle is not one
of the reasons. We are also suspicious when an epidemiologist doth
protest too much. Protein is chemically complex; or more precisely,
there are hundreds of different proteins that might have opposite
effects in the body. There are twenty amino acids that make up these
proteins and they, in turn, have many individual effects and some work

together with the others. We are asked to believe that after they are digested, our bodies can tell which amino acids came from animals and which from vegetables.

It is not even clear that most of us eat a lot of meat. Protein tends to be a stable part of the diet. There was no change in protein consumption in the last forty years during the period of the obesity and diabetes epidemic. We might eat more than recommended by health agencies, but their credentials are up for renewal. In fact many individuals, particularly the elderly, don't get enough meat. Given the complexities, it seems that the burden of proof should be on those who want to show the dangers of meat. Both the scientific and popular press, however, give you the idea that meat should be considered guilty until proven innocent.

Red meat, in particular, is "linked to" just about every disease imaginable, including diabetes, where if anything, it is likely to be beneficial. The lipophobes' approach is epidemiological and their numerous papers have a common theme: find a weak association and claim that if the risk, no matter how miniscule, is multiplied by the whole population, we can save thousands of lives by reducing meat consumption. Here, again, I am asking you to accept the idea that the best and the brightest are not doing acceptable science. Using the principles from the previous chapters, I will analyze a couple of specific papers. These reports provide examples of the particular errors that you can look for when trying to decide if a scientific paper is valid or not.

One important idea: All of statistics is subjective. Assumptions are made and numbers are calculated from those assumptions. The numbers are meaningful only if the assumptions fit the question to be answered. You have to remember that statistical significance is a mathematical term, meaning that differences between an experimental group and the controls in a particular experiment did not arise by chance. It does not mean, however, that those differences are of sufficient magnitude or are of sufficient reliability that if the experiment were repeated it would not turn out differently. It does not mean that the differences have any practical or clinical significance, either. I'll begin with an older red meat study, which illustrates the limitations of relative risk and odds ratios. This particular case has a punch line, and I'll show you that the whole paper was probably some kind of flimflam.

Red Meat Scare of 2009

"Daily Red Meat Raises Chances of Dying Early" was the headline in the March 24, 2009, issue of the *Washington Post*.[2] This scare story was accompanied by a photo of a gloved hand slicing beef with a scalpel-like knife, probably intended to evoke a *CSI* autopsy (although it still looked pretty good to me, if slightly overcooked). I don't know the reporter, Rob Stein, but I don't think we're talking about anyone on the level of Woodward and Bernstein. For those too young to remember Watergate, the reporters from the *Post* were encouraged to "follow the money" by Deep Throat, their anonymous whistleblower. The movie *Fat Head* suggests the variation —more appropriate here—that we "follow the data."

In the strange world of nutrition, scandalous behavior is right out in the open. Researchers don't like to be whistleblowers, because unless the issue has some major impact, a breakdown in research principles makes us all look bad. The missteps in published papers in nutrition, however, require no insider information to pick apart. The *Washington Post* story was based on a study, "Meat Intake and Mortality," published in the professional medical journal *Archives of Internal Medicine* by Rashmi Sinha and coauthors.[3] It got a certain amount of press at the time of publication, but following the usual pattern, it soon disappeared from view into the pile of "accumulating evidence" that meat would kill you. Nobody looked at it closely. Certainly not Rob Stein. To be fair, it's not his fault. It takes time to analyze such papers and he was likely assigned to a flower show the next day. Although it is not unreasonable that he took the authors at their word, it is worth looking at the details now. When analyzing studies on the risk of a diet or drugs, looking back to Bradford Hill's criteria, we should expect that there first be specificity. (Recall how Hill emphasized that it was lung and nose cancer specifically that were associated with cigarette smoking.) However, specificity is exactly what was lacking in Sinha et al.'s paper, whose main outcome measure was all-cause mortality—that is, the number of deaths from *any* disease. If a paper is about all-cause mortality, then the check on specificity is lost and we should be sure that this is for real. Unsurprisingly, the conclusion will be that the paper fails to make a good case for the danger of red meat, and in fact, its greatest virtue may be in showing you how to see through the flaws that populate the literature.

Common Sense and Experience First

Your best bet in dealing with potential bias is to demand that, no matter how complicated the statistics are, the results should not violate common sense—or if they do seem to be counterintuitive, that they are convincingly justified. The further the conclusion deviates from common sense or previous established results, the greater the demand for that justification. The salient fact about red meat

Principle 1

Biology, common sense, and experience come before statistics. Do the results make sense?

is that during the thirty years that we describe as the obesity and diabetes epidemic, overall protein intake was relatively constant, and red meat consumption actually went down by a significant degree. As previously shown in chapter 1, almost all of the caloric increase in that period was due to an increase in carbohydrates. Fat, if anything, went down. However, during this period, consumption of almost everything else went up: Wheat and corn, of course, skyrocketed, but so did fruits and vegetables. The two notable foods whose consumption went down were red meat and eggs. In addition, we need to remember that much research shows the benefits of replacing carbohydrate with protein, especially for the elderly.[4] So, here's something that you can use as a rule in analyzing papers in the literature.

Simple Statistics: Who's Likely to Die?

The paper by Rashmi Sinha et al.[5] is an observational study of the type discussed in the previous chapter: They tried to match outcomes for different groups in an existing population with their dietary behavior. In terms of informing the public, the report in the *Washington Post* is quite a bit more accessible than the original paper. It reads:

> Researchers analyzed data from 545,653 predominantly white volunteers, ages 50 to 71, participating in the National Institutes

of Health-AARP Diet and Health Study. In 1995, the subjects filled out detailed questionnaires about their diets, including meat consumption. Over the next 10 years, 47,976 men and 23,276 women died.

So the risk, or probability, of dying if you were in the study population is easy to calculate from the *Washington Post* report: overall probability = (number of people who died) / (all the people in the study). That is equal to (47,976 + 23, 276)/545,653 = 0.13 or 13 percent. This is a good reference point, something that we're sure of before anybody starts doing the statistics. The risk is not

Principle 2

Are the results meaningful— that is, large numbers?

great. Only slightly more than one in ten people died in the course of the experiment. The article goes on to say:

> Those who ate the most red meat—about a quarter-pound a day—were more likely to die of any reason, and from heart disease and cancer in particular, than those who ate the least— the equivalent of a couple of slices of ham a day. Among women, those who ate the most red meat were 36 percent more likely to die for any reason, 20 percent more likely to die of cancer and 50 percent more likely to die of heart disease. Men who ate the most meat were 31 percent more likely to die for any reason, 22 percent more likely to die of cancer and 27 percent more likely to die of heart disease.

That sounds fairly scary, but is it? By this point you might be experiencing an emotional reaction to relative risk. This is almost always misleading. So, let's do what scientists call a back-of-the-envelope calculation to see if we can get meaningful numbers. You can skip this if you don't like math, but it's really not bad—just high school algebra. We have the overall risk of mortality: 13 percent. Now, for both men and women, the increase in risk from eating meat is about 33 percent (36 percent for women; 31 percent for men), so if N people died in the low-meat group, then $1.33N$ died among the high-meat group. Together they make up 13 percent of the total, so we have: $(N + 1.33N) = 2.33N = 13$ percent. If you solve for N you get 0.0558, or about 5.6 percent. From there we can determine that the risk in the low-meat group is 5.6 percent, and the risk in the high-meat group is 7.4 percent. So the absolute difference in risk is only 1.8 percent. Before you even look at the original paper, we are now talking about a difference in risk in the ballpark of a few percent. Your steak is already sounding a lot better.

What we are trying to do here is to go beyond relative risk and get at absolute risk. The dire warning that "those who ate the most red meat were 36 percent more likely to die for any reason" lost its kick when we did an absolute risk calculation. Why? Obviously, when it is a case of relative anything, you need to know: Relative to what? In diseases with low prevalence, or events with low probability, relative risk is almost always misleading.

What Was Measured?

Another problem is that the paper says "A 124-item food frequency questionnaire . . . was completed at baseline." Many are suspicious of food questionnaires because people might not accurately report what they ate. While this can be a source of error, the amount of error depends on how the data is interpreted. All scientific measurements have error. Here the problem is the word "baseline." The study was started in 1995, continued for ten years, and mortality was followed during this period. This means that some people died as long as ten years after their reported food intake. The take-home question here: Are you eating the same thing you were eating ten years ago? More to the point, with all the kvetching about red meat in the media, is there a chance somebody in this study reduced red meat consumption? Is there a chance that they did it halfway through the study and would have appeared in a different group if data had been collected for them at that halfway point? To simplify even further: If I get sick, it is due to the junk I ate in college?

But, let's take them at their word and assume the study is okay. What do we learn from the outcome? The damned statistics, as Mark Twain might have called them, go like this: The study population of 322,263 men and 223,390 women was broken up into five groups (quintiles) according to meat consumption, with the highest group taking in about seven times as much as the lowest group. The groups were compared according to a statistic called hazard ratio (HR), which, as explained below, in cases like this is more or less the same as relative risk. The authors report that the HR for eating red meat every day compared to eating red meat rarely is 1.44. This is pretty weak. Before discussing further, I'll explain the different terms for expressing risk. Again, the math is simple, but you can skip ahead if you're daunted.

Understanding OR, RR, and HR

The common measures of relative outcomes in comparing a nutritional or medical intervention with controls are odds ratio (OR), relative risk (RR), and hazard ratio (HR). The good news is that for most of the studies relevant to what we're doing here, these statistical measures are all pretty much the same (because the incidence of disease or other outcome is low). As described above, "risk" in medicine is the probability of a given outcome, and relative risk is what it sounds like—the probability of an outcome occurring in one group compared to the probability of it occurring in a second group.

> **Principle 3**
>
> If the effect is not large, then the data have to be very reliable. Conversely, if the data have big potential error, then the conclusion must be substantial.

Let's break things down. Probability is equal to the number of particular outcomes divided by the total number of possible outcomes. We can look at some examples from the world of gambling, using the word *winning* as a stand-in for any particular outcome, such as getting sick or losing a target amount of weight:

Probability = Number of ways of winning/Total possible outcomes

Probability of drawing an ace from a fair deck = 4 aces/52 total cards = 1/13 = 0.0769

Probability of drawing the ace of spades from a fair deck = 1 ace of spades/52 total cards = 1/52 = 0.0192

In some cases, rather than the probability, the odds might be reported. Odds are slightly different from probability:

Odds = Number of ways of winning/Number of ways of not winning

Odds of drawing an ace from a fair deck = 4 aces/48 non-aces cards = 1/12 = 0.0833

Odds of drawing the ace of spades from a fair deck = 1 ace of spades / 51 non-ace of spades cards = 1/51 = 0.0196

As the likelihood of an event occurring diminishes, the odds and the probability move closer together and are used similarly in conversation. This is evident in the examples above: The probability of drawing the ace of spades from a fair deck is 1 out of 52, or .0192, while the odds are 1 out of 51, or .0196. Because the event is unlikely to occur, the difference between odds and probability becomes almost negligible.

In an experiment comparing outcomes between two groups, for example cancer in meat eaters and cancer in vegetarians, you might report relative risk (RR):

Relative Risk = (Probability of an outcome in group 1) / (Probability of outcome in group 2)

Relative risk of drawing any ace, compared to drawing an ace of spades:

(4/54) / (1/54) = 4

In a medical experiment you might not be able to wait until the experiment is over to calculate the probability of a given outcome. This is where hazard comes into play. Hazard is the same as the probability, but measured over fixed time intervals. For example, you might measure how many people get sick in the first month in each group in a study. Hazard is a rate and is the probability of "winning" for a fixed time period. There is slightly more to hazard, mathematically, but in most papers it is reported as the hazard ratio (HR) between two interventions. The bottom line in these cases is that you can think of HR as the same as RR.

It is important to realize that once you calculate RR, HR, or OR, you have lost track of how much absolute risk there was to begin with. If a paper tells you the RR of a disease, you don't know whether it is a rare disease or one that everybody has. Bottom line: In reading a scientific paper, you can take RR, HR, and OR as roughly the same. They all provide a comparison between how likely two events are to occur. The big caveat is that you have to make sure you know what the individual probability of each event is. The problem is described well in the following narrative.

You are in Las Vegas. There are two blackjack tables, and for some reason they have different probabilities of paying out (different number of decks, for example). The probability of winning at Table One is 1 in 100 hands, or 1 percent. At Table Two the probability of winning is 1 in 80 hands, or about 1.27 percent. The ratio of the probabilities (RR of winning) is 1.27 / 1.0 = 1.27. (A ratio of 1 would mean that there is no difference between the tables.) Suppose all that you know is the RR of 1.27. Right off, something is wrong: You are missing a lot of information. One gambling table is definitely better than the other, but you have no way of knowing whether the odds at either table are particularly good in the first place.

Suppose, however, that you did get a glimpse at the real info and you could find out what the absolute odds are at the different tables: 1 percent at Table One and 1.27 percent at Table Two. Does that help? Well, it depends on who you are. For the guy who is sitting at the black-jack table when you go up to sleep in your room at the hotel, and who is still there when you come down for the breakfast buffet, he is going to be much better off at Table Two. He will play hundreds of hands and the slightly better odds ratio of 1.27 is likely to pay off. On the other hand, imagine that you are somebody who will take the advice of my cousin, the statistician, who says to just go and play one hand for the fun of it, just to see if the universe loves you (that's what gamblers are really trying to find out). You're going to play the hand, win or lose, and then go off and do something else. Does it matter which table you play at? Obviously it doesn't. The odds ratio doesn't tell you anything useful because your chances of winning are pretty slim either way.

Differences in Absolute Risk

Returning to the original red meat paper, there are a number of different "models" (reworking of the data) and there are mind-numbing tables giving you the different hazard ratios. Using the worst case HR between high and low red meat intakes for men, we get HR = 1.48, or, as they like to report in the media, 48 percent higher risk of dying from all causes. It sounds bad, but wait: What is the absolute difference in risk? Well, the paper says that the whole group of 322,263 men was divided into five subgroups (quintiles) of 64,453 people each. (Note that you usually have to dig this information out of tables. Authors don't always make it easy to find the data, which is itself cause for suspicion.) The people who don't eat much red meat had 6,437 deaths, or 10.0 percent by population. The big meat eaters must then have had 14.8 percent deaths. That's an absolute difference of only 5 percent. The authors then corrected for some things that might have contributed to the outcome, bringing the absolute difference for men down to a mere 3 percent.

Bottom line: There is an absolute difference in risk of about 3 percent. It is unreasonable to think that this represents a call to change your life. Remember, too, that this is for big changes—like six or seven times as much meat. So, what is a meaningful HR? For comparison, the HR for smoking versus not smoking, with regard to lung disease, was about 20. For heavy smokers, the HR was about 30. Going back to Bradford Hill's criteria: "First upon my list I would put the strength of the association." Relative risk does not have meaning by itself. You must know the changes in absolute risk. Another common way of looking at the data that is more meaningful is the number needed to treat (NNT), which is the reciprocal of the absolute risk. For our 3 percent risk in Sinha's red meat study, you would have to treat twenty to thirty people to save one life. That's not great but it's something. Or is it?

What About Public Health? Good News or Not?

Many people would say that, sure, for a single person, red meat might not make a difference, but if the population reduced meat by half, we could save thousands of lives. At this point, before you and your family take part in a big experiment to save health statistics in the country, you have to apply Principles 2 and 3. You have to ask how strong the relations are, and to understand how good the data is, you must look for things that would not be expected to have a correlation. "There was an increased risk associated with death from injuries and sudden death with higher consumption of red meat in men but not in women," which sounds like we are dealing with a good deal of randomness.

More important, what is the risk in reducing meat intake? The data don't really tell you that. Unlike cigarettes, where there is little reason to believe that anybody's lungs benefit from cigarette smoke, we know that there are many benefits to protein, especially if it replaces carbohydrate in the diet, especially for the elderly, and especially for all kinds of people. So with odds ratios around 1, you are almost as likely to benefit from adding red meat as you are reducing it. Technically, it is called a two-tailed distribution, which is to say that things can change in both directions. The odds still favor things getting worse but it is a risk in both directions. You are at the gaming tables. You don't get your chips back. If you bet on reducing red meat and it does not reduce your risk, it will increase your risk.

The Fine Print: The Smoking Gun

In writing this chapter, which was based on a blog post, I went back to the original paper to check the calculations. I had used the numbers for men because it was a worst case (and it still has the problems that I described), but in recalculating things, I looked at the numbers for women as well. The data unfolded like this.

The population was again broken up into five groups, or quintiles. The lower numbered quintiles are for the lowest consumption of red meat. Looking at the reported data on all-cause mortality, there were 5,314 deaths for low consumption. When you go up to quintile 5—that is, highest red meat consumption—there are 3,752 deaths. What? The more red meat, the lower the death rate? In other words, the raw data show the opposite of the conclusion of the paper. There were fewer deaths at high red meat. The confounders are listed in the legend to the figure. For the "basic model," the data were corrected for race and total energy intake, and risk went up. Why? We can't tell if we can't see what the effect was. Do you have the sense of flimflam?

A useful way to look at this data is from the standpoint of conditional probability. We ask: What is the probability of dying in this experiment if you consume a high-meat diet? The answer is simply the number of people who both died during the experiment and were big meat-eaters (Q5) divided by the total number of individuals in Q5. Here's the calculation: $3{,}752/(223{,}3905) = 0.0839$, or about 8 percent. If you are not a big meat-eater, your risk is $(5{,}314 + 5{,}081 + 4{,}734 + 4{,}395)/(0.8 \times 223{,}390) = 0.109$, or about 11 percent.

This paper tested the hypothesis that red meat is associated with all-cause mortality. The data showed that it wasn't. Meat wasn't a risk unless you dragged in other factors: education, marital status, family history of cancer, body mass index, smoking history using smoking status (never, former, current), time since quitting for former smokers, physical activity, alcohol intake, vitamin supplement user, fruit consumption, and vegetable consumption. All of these have to be added in to make the authors' conclusion true. Once you do that, though, you have to ask why you would single out red meat among these other ten inputs as the key variable. Wouldn't it be better to find out which of these factors had the biggest effect? What I offer here is a professional scientist's view, and I try to make my description dispassionate and not insulting, but what is this if not deception?

What Is It About Red Meat?

Red meat isn't a chemical, so what is it about the red meat that upsets people? The meat? The red? To be fair to the authors, they also studied white meat, which they found by the same prestidigitation mostly beneficial. But what about potatoes? Cupcakes? Breakfast cereal? Are these completely neutral? If we ran all these factors through the same computer, what would we see? Unspoken in everybody's mind is saturated fat, that Rasputin of nutritional risk factors who will come after you despite enough bullets in its body to have killed several scientific theories. Maybe it wasn't the red meat per se but the way it was procured. Maybe it's ritual slaughter that conferred eternal life (or lack of it) on the consumer. For a gripping description of the total spiritual effect of bad behavior, nothing is as harrowing as the Isaac Bashevis Singer stories equating meat eating with other sins of the flesh. Finally, there is the elephant in the room: carbohydrate. Basic biochemistry suggests that a roast beef sandwich might have a different effect than roast beef in a lettuce wrap.

The Right Questions

My hope is that you will come away from this chapter with some basic rules for dealing with the scientific literature—questions to ask and principles to apply:

1. Do the results make sense? Biology comes before statistics. Experience comes before statistics.
2. Is there a big association? Are we talking about meaningful, that is, large numbers?
3. What was measured? If the effect is not large, then the data have to be very reliable. If the data have big potential error, then the conclusion must be substantial.

In nutrition, as in other fields, recommendations are often tinged by the personal preferences of those dishing them out. In combination with the dogmatic state of government and private recommendations, it takes some work to know if you are reading a meaningful study. The point of this chapter, and of this entire section of the book, is that you have the right to ask for, and the author has the obligation to provide, clear explanations. The practical application of Hill's criteria is that results should make sense in terms of magnitude and what you know about biology. You should also be very suspicious if only relative risk is reported, even if just in the Abstract. Remember, Alice has 30 percent more money in the bank than Bob, but we don't know whether she is rich.

You can usually calculate absolute risk (the number of cases divided by the number of participants) so you can see if the report is about something that is very rare. The specific case in this chapter, the effect of red meat, fails to meet the criterion of meaningful associations and seems to be deployed to distract from the real culprit, the real elephant in the room: carbohydrate.

Harvard:
Making Americans Afraid of Red Meat

"There was a sense of déjà-vu about the paper by Pan, et al. entitled 'Red meat consumption and mortality: results from 2 prospective cohort studies'[6] that came out in April of 2012." That's what I wrote online in May of 2012. Other bloggers worked it over pretty well, so I ignored the paper for the most part. Then I came across a remarkable article from the Harvard Health Blog. Titled "Study Urges Moderation in Red Meat Intake," it was about the Pan et al. study and it described how the "study linking red meat and mortality lit up the media." It claimed that "headline writers had a field day, with entries like 'Red meat death study,' 'Will red meat kill you?' and 'Singing the blues about red meat.'" This was too much for me.

What was odd about the post from the Harvard blog was that "the field day for headline writers" was all described from a distance, as if the study by Pan et al. (and the content of the Harvard blogpost itself) hadn't come from Harvard, but was rather a natural phenomenon, similar to the way every seminar on obesity begins with a graphic of the state-by-state progression of obesity as if it were some kind of meteorological event.

The reference to "headline writers," I think, was intended to conjure images of sleazy tabloid publishers like the ones who are always pushing the limits of First Amendment rights in the old *Law & Order* episodes. The Harvard blogpost itself, however, was not any less exaggerated. It is not true that the Harvard study urged moderation. In fact, the article admitted that the original paper "sounded ominous. Every extra daily serving of unprocessed red meat (steak, hamburger, pork, etc.) increased the risk of dying prematurely by 13%. Processed red meat (hot dogs, sausage, bacon, and the like) upped the risk by 20%."

That is what the paper urged. Not moderation. Prohibition. "Increased the risk of dying prematurely by 13%." Who wants to buck odds like that? Who wants to die prematurely?

It wasn't just the media. Critics in the blogosphere were also working overtime deconstructing the study. Among the faults cited was the reporting of relative risk. Once again: Relative risk is relative. It doesn't tell you what the risk is to begin with. Relative risk destroys information. The extreme example remains that you can double your odds of winning the lottery if you buy two tickets instead of one. So why do people keep reporting it? One reason, of course, is that it makes your work look more significant than it is, but if you don't report the absolute change in risk, you might be scaring people about risks that aren't real. The nutritional establishment is not good at facing their critics, but in this case, Harvard admitted that they didn't wish to push back against their detractors.

Nolo Contendere
Having turned the media loose to scare the American public, Harvard admitted that the bloggers were correct. The Harvard Health Blog allocuted to having reported "relative risks, comparing death rates in the group eating the least meat with those eating the most." "The absolute risks," they admitted, "sometimes help tell the story a bit more clearly. These numbers are somewhat less scary." Why not try to tell the story as clearly as possible in the original article then?

Anyway, there was a table on the Harvard Health Blog that presented the raw data. This is what you need to know. Unfortunately, the Harvard Health Blog didn't actually calculate the absolute risk for you. You'd think that they would want to make up for Dr. Pan scaring you. After all, an allocution is supposed to remove doubt about the details of the crimes. Let's calculate the absolute risk. It's not hard.

As previously, risk is a probability: that is, number of cases divided by total number of participants. Looking at the data for the men first, the risk of death with three servings per week is equal to 12.3 cases per 1,000 people, or 1.23 percent. Now going to fourteen servings a week the risk of death is 13 cases per 1,000, or 1.3 percent. So, for men, the absolute difference in risk is less than 0.1 percent. Definitely less scary. In fact, not scary at all.

Still, at least according to the public health professionals, the risk could add up for millions of people. Or could it? We have to step back and ask what is predictable about showing a change of less than one-tenth of 1 percent risk. It means that a small unpredictable event—a couple of guys getting hit by cars in one or another of the groups—might throw the whole thing off (remember we're talking total deaths). Many other things have a lower risk than that, but might not have been considered. Maybe a handful of guys in upscale, vegetarian social circles lied about their late night trips to Dinosaur Barbecue. The number has no real-world significance. When can you scale up a small outcome? If the outcome number is small, and you want to scale it up, it must be secure and have little room for error.

There is an underlying theme here. There is the possibility that the mass of epidemiology studies from the Harvard School of Public Health and other groups are simply not real. Poor understanding of science, cognitive dissonance, or something else altogether might be the cause. Whatever it is, the progression of epidemiologic studies showing that meat causes diabetes, that sugar causes gout, all with low-hazard ratios—that is, small association size—might be meaningless. It's discouraging and almost impossible to believe. A big piece of medical research is a house of cards.

Who Paid for This and What Should Be Done

We paid for it. Pan et al. were funded in part by six National Institutes of Health grants and NIH is still paying for it. The latest production from this group now emphasizes the "change in meat consumption."[7] Remarkably, my objections to this paper were published as a letter to the editor.[8] My main point was that "Red meat consumption decreased as T2DM [type 2 diabetes mellitus] increased during the past 30 years."

It is hard to believe with all the flaws pointed out by myself and others, and in the end, admitted by the Harvard Health Blog, that this work was subject to any meaningful peer review. A plea of no contest does not imply negligence or intent to do harm, but something is wrong. There is the clear attempt to influence the dietary habits of the population. This cannot sensibly be justified by an absolute risk reduction of less than one-tenth of 1 percent, especially given that others have made the case that some part of the population, particularly the elderly, might not get adequate protein. The need for an oversight committee of impartial scientists is the most reasonable conclusion from Pan et al.

CHAPTER 15

The Seventh Egg

When Studies Defy Common Sense

S tepping back and looking at the recent nutritional literature, I am struck by the miracle of life. How could humans have evolved in the face of threats from red meat, eggs, and even shaving? (The Caerphilly Prospective Study shows you the dangers of shaving . . . or is it the dangers of not shaving?[1]) With 28 percent greater risk of diabetes here and 57 percent greater risk of heart disease there, how could our ancestors ever have come of childbearing age? Considering the daily revelations from the Harvard School of Public Health, showing the Scylla of saturated fat and the Charybdis of sugar between which our forefathers sailed, it is a miracle that we're here.

These sensational stories that the popular media writes about, are they real? They are, after all, based on scientific papers. Although not all members of the media have the expertise to decipher them, reporters generally talk to the researchers—and the papers must have gone through peer review in the first place, right? However, as the previous chapters suggest, the gatekeepers, as we think of peer reviewers, are less vigilant than they should be. In fact, many papers that are published in the major medical journals defy common sense. While it is hard to believe, the medical literature really does have a remarkably high degree of error. Medical publications are burdened with many examples of misinterpretation and poor understanding of scientific design and analysis. While there is little outright falsification of data, the researchers are not always doing credible science. How can the consumer decide?

I am going to illustrate the problem with the example of a paper by L. Djoussé: "Egg Consumption and Risk of Type 2 Diabetes in Men and Women."[2] In the study by Djoussé et al., participants were asked how many eggs they ate and then, ten years later, it was determined whether they had developed diabetes. If they had, it was assumed to be because of the number of eggs. Is this for real? Do eggs really cause changes in your body that accumulate until you develop a disease—a disease that is, after all, primarily one of carbohydrate intolerance? Type 2 diabetes, recall, is due to impaired response of the body to the insulin produced by beta cells of the pancreas, as well as a progressive deterioration of the insulin-producing cells. Common sense tells us it's unlikely that eggs could play a major role, but it is still important to understand the methodology and see if there is a something that justifies this obvious departure from common sense. Again, Hill's principles might be useful.

What did the experimenters actually do? First, subjects were specifically asked "to report how often, on average, they had eaten one egg during the past year," and subjects where thus classified into one the following categories of egg consumption: 0, <1 per week, 1 per week, 2–4 per week, 5–6 per week, and 7+ eggs per week. The researchers collected these data every other year for ten years. With these data in hand, they then followed subjects "from baseline until the first occurrence of one of the following: (a) diagnosis of type 2 diabetes; (b) death; or (c) censoring date, the date of receipt of the last follow-up questionnaire," which for men was up to twenty years.

Take a second and consider the last year of your life. Is it possible that you might not be able to remember whether you had one versus two eggs per week on average during the year? Is there any possibility that some of the subjects who were diagnosed with diabetes ten years after their report on egg consumption had changed their eating pattern over the course of that decade-long experiment? Are you eating the same food you ate ten years ago? Quick, how many eggs per week did you eat last year?

The Golden Rule Again

Right off, there is a problem in people accurately reporting what they ate. This is a limitation of many—probably most—nutritional studies, and while it can be a source of error, it is really a question of how you interpret the data. All scientific measurements have error. You simply have to be sure that the results that you are trying to find do not depend on any greater accuracy than the data that you have collected. Eyeballing the paper by

Djoussé et al., we see that there are no figures, which is already a suspicious sign. We would have expected, at least, a graph of the number of eggs consumed versus the number of cases of diabetes. The results, instead, are stated in the abstract of the paper in the form of this mind-numbing conclusion (don't actually try to read this; it is merely an illustration of the tedious writing in the medical literature):

> Compared with no egg consumption, multivariable adjusted hazard ratios (95% CI) for type 2 diabetes were 1.09 (0.87–1.37), 1.09 (0.88–1.34), 1.18 (0.95–1.45), 1.46 (1.14–1.86), and 1.58 (1.25–2.01) for consumption of <1, 1, 2–4, 5–6, and 7+ eggs/ week, respectively, in men (p for trend <0.0001). Corresponding multivariable hazard ratios (95% CI) for women were 1.06 (0.92–1.22), 0.97 (0.83–1.12), 1.19 (1.03–1.38), 1.18 (0.88– 1.58), and 1.77 (1.28–2.43), respectively (p for trend <0.0001).

What does all this mean? Very little. These "statistical shenanigans" are, in fact, an argument against a correlation. If you look at the paragraph, almost every number that you see is very close to 1. Without going through a detailed analysis, you can simply extract from the tables some simple information: There were 1,921 men who developed diabetes. Of these, 197 were in the high egg consumption group, or about 10 percent. For women, there were 2,112 cases of diabetes, of whom 46 were high egg consumers, or a little more than 2 percent. To me this suggests that diabetes is associated with something other than eggs, and that it is probably unjustified of the authors to conclude: "These data suggest that high levels of egg consumption (daily) are associated with an increased risk of type 2 diabetes in men and women."

What I described are the raw data, and as we saw in chapter 14, we have to consider confounders. In fact, if we analyzed the data in detail, we would find that the conclusion is actually poorly supported by the data, but let's take the authors' conclusion at face value for the sake of argument.

The Seventh Egg

If the authors' conclusion is correct, this means that there was no additional risk of diabetes from consuming 1 egg per week as compared to eating none. Similarly, there was no additional risk in eating 2–4 eggs per week or 5–6 eggs per week. However if you upped your intake to 7 eggs or more per week, then that's it: You were at risk for diabetes. It makes me think of the movie *The Seventh Seal*, directed by Ingmar Bergman. Very popular in the fifties and sixties, these movies had a captivating if pretentious style: They sometimes seemed to be designed for the Woody Allen's parodies that would follow. One of the famous scenes in *The Seventh Seal* is the protagonist's chess game with Death. It requires only a little imagination to see the egg as the incarnation of the Grim Reaper.

Mindless Statistics

A study of 20,703 men and 36,295 women makes a very weak case for a connection between egg consumption and type 2 diabetes. Few of the people who developed diabetes were big egg eaters. The problem is the mindless use of statistics. If statistics ever go against common sense, it is the authors' responsibility to explain why—in detail and in the abstract.

Sometimes, you can get a sense of how real the statistics are by looking for simple things: How many people were in the study and how many got sick? In other words, are we talking about a rare disease or one that had low probability? In the case of this particular experiment from Djoussé et al., diabetes is a major health risk, but if you take 1,000 men for ten years, and only 1 in 10 might develop diabetes, you need to be sure there is a big difference between the group that followed the behavior you are looking at (egg consumption) and those who didn't.

CHAPTER 16

Intention-to-Treat

What It Is and Why You Should Care

The medical literature has some strange customs, but nothing beats intention-to-treat (ITT), the most absurd and amusing statistical method that has appeared recently. According to ITT, the data from a subject assigned at random to an experimental group must be included in the reported outcome data for that group, even if the subject does not follow the protocol, or even if they drop out of the experiment. In other words, it doesn't matter if you eat what the experimenter told you to eat—your lipid profile has to be included in the final report. It's easy enough to tell that the idea is counterintuitive if not completely idiotic—why would you include people who are not in the experiment in your data? The burden of proof in using such a method should rest with its proponents, but no such obligation is felt, and particularly in nutrition studies—such as comparisons of isocaloric weight-loss diets—ITT is frequently used with no justification at all. Astoundingly, the practice is sometimes actually demanded by reviewers in the scientific journals. As one might expect, there is a good deal of controversy on this subject. Physiologists or chemists, or really anybody with scientific training, who hears about ITT requirements will usually walk away shaking their head or uttering some obvious *reductio ad absurdum*—for instance, "You mean, if nobody takes the pill, you report whether or not they got better anyway?" That's exactly what it means. In this chapter I'll describe a couple of interesting cases from the medical literature, and one relatively new instance—Foster's two-year study of low-carbohydrate diets—to demonstrate the abuse of common sense that is the major characteristic of ITT.

On the naïve assumption that some people really didn't understand what was wrong with ITT—I've been known to make a few elementary mistakes in my life—I wrote a paper on the subject. It received negative, even hostile, reviews from two public health journals. I even got substantial grief from reviewers at *Nutrition and Metabolism*, where it was finally published. I was the editor at the time, and I had extensive communications with one reviewer who was willing to forego anonymity.

The title of my paper was "Intention-to-Treat. What Is the Question?" My point was that there's nothing inherently wrong with ITT if you are explicit about what you are measuring. If you use ITT, you are really asking: What is the effect of assigning subjects to an experimental protocol? However, is anybody really interested in what the patient was told to do rather than what they actually did?

The practice of ITT comes from clinical trials, where you can't always tell whether patients have taken the recommended pills, just as in the real situation where you never know what people will do once they leave the doctor's office. In that case you do an analysis based on your intention; that is, you have no other choice than to designate those who were assigned to the intervention as the "experimental group," even though they might not have participated in the experiment. That's what we always did without giving it a special name. When you do know who took the pill and who didn't, however, there are two separate questions: Did they take the pill, and is the pill any good? That's the data. You have to know both, and if you want to collapse them into one number, you have to be sure you make clear what you are talking about. You lose information if you collapse efficacy and adherence into one number. It is common for the abstract of a paper to correctly state that the results are about subjects "assigned to a diet" but by the time the results are presented, the independent variable has usually become simply "the diet," rather than "assignment to diet," which most people would assume meant what people ate rather than what they were told to eat. *Caveat lector.*

My paper on ITT was perhaps overkill. I made several different arguments, but a single commonsense argument gets to the heart of the problem. I'll describe that first, along with a couple of real-world examples.

Commonsense Argument Against Intention-to-Treat

Consider an experimental comparison of two diets in which there is a simple, discrete outcome (e.g., a threshold amount of weight lost or

Table 16.1. Hypothetical Results from the Thought Experiment for Analysis of Diets A and B

	Diet A	Diet B
Compliance (of 100 patients)	50	100
Success (reached target)	50	50
ITT success	50/100 = 50%	50/100 = 50%
"Per protocol" (followed diet) success	50/50 = 100%	50/100 = 50%

remission of an identifiable symptom.) Patients are randomly assigned to two different diets, diet A or diet B, and a target of, say, 5 kilograms of weight loss is considered success. As shown in table 16.1, half of the subjects in diet A are "compliers," able to stay on the diet, while the other half are not. The half of the patients on diet A who were compliers were all able to lose the target 5 kilograms, while the noncompliers did not. In diet B, on the other hand, everybody stayed on the diet, but somehow only half were able to lose the required amount of weight. An ITT analysis shows no difference in the two outcomes—half of group A stayed on the diet and all lost weight, while in study B, everybody complied but only half had success.

Now, suppose you are the doctor. With such data in hand, should you advise a patient: "Well, the diets are pretty much the same. It's largely up to you which you choose," as required by ITT? Or, alternatively, looking at the raw data would the recommendation be: "Diet A is much more effective than diet B, but people have trouble staying on it. If you can stay on diet A, it will be much better for you, so I would encourage you to see if you could find a way to do so." You are the doctor. Which makes more sense?

Diet A is obviously better, but it's hard for people to stay on it. This is one of the characteristics of ITT: It always makes the better diet look worse than it is. In the submitted manuscript, I made several arguments trying to explain that there are two factors. One of them, whether it actually works, is directly due to the diet. The other, whether you follow the diet, is under control of other factors (whether WebMD tells you that one diet or the other will kill you, whether the evening news makes you lose your appetite, etc.). I even dragged in a geometric argument because Newton had used one in the *Principia*: "A two-dimensional outcome space where the length of a vector tells how every subject did . . . ITT represents a projection of the vector onto one axis, in other words collapses a two-dimensional vector to a one-dimensional vector, thereby losing part of the information." Pretentious? *Moi?*

Why You Should Care: Surgery or Medicine?

Does your doctor actually read these academic studies using ITT? One can only hope not. Consider the analysis by David Newell of the Coronary Artery Bypass Surgery (CABS) trial. This paper is fascinating for the blanket, tendentious insistence, without any logical argument, on something that is obviously fundamentally foolish. Newell wrote: "The CABS research team was impeccable. They refused to do an 'as treated' analysis: We have refrained from comparing all patients actually operated on with all not operated on: This does not provide a measure of the value of surgery."[1]

You read it right. The results of surgery do not provide a measure of the value of surgery.

In the CABS trial, patients were assigned to be treated with either medicine or surgery. The actual method used and the outcomes are shown in table 16.2. Looking at the table, you see the effects of assignments (ITT): 7.8 percent mortality for those *assigned* to receive medical treatment (29 deaths out of 373), and 5.3 percent mortality for those assigned to surgery (21 deaths of 371). On the other hand if you look at the *outcomes* of each treatment as actually used, it turns out that medical treatment had a mortality rate of 9.5 percent (33 deaths of 349), while among those who

Table 16.2. Results from the CABS Trial from Newell

	Allocated medicine		Allocated surgery	
	Received surgery	Received medicine	Received surgery	Received medicine
Survived 2 years	48	296	354	20
Died	2	27	15	6
Total	50	323	369	26

Source: David J. Newell, "Intention-to-Treat Analysis: Implications for Quantitative and Qualitative Research," *International Journal of Epidemiology* 23, no. 5 (1992): 837–841.

actually underwent surgery, the mortality rate was only 4.1 percent (17 deaths of 419). Mortality was less than half in surgery compared to medical treatment. Making such a simple statement, that surgery was better than medicine, Newell claimed, "would have wildly exaggerated the apparent value of surgery." The "apparent value of surgery"? Common sense suggests that appearances are not deceiving. If you were one of the 16 people who were still alive because you chose surgery based on outcome (17 deaths) rather than because of ITT (33 deaths), you would think that it was the theoretical report of your death that had been exaggerated.

The thing that is under the control of the patient and the physician, and that is not a feature of the particular modality, is getting the surgery actually done. Common sense dictates that a patient is interested in surgery, not the effect of being told that surgery is good. The patient has a right to expect that if they comply with the recommendation for surgery, the physician should try to avoid any mistakes from previous studies that prevented other patients from actually receiving the operation. In another defense of ITT, Hollis and Campbell made the somewhat cryptic statement: "Most types of deviations from protocol would continue to occur in routine practice."[2] This seems to be saying that the same number of people will always forget to take their medication and surgeons will continue to have exactly the same scheduling problems as in the CABS trial. ITT assumes that practical considerations are the same everywhere and that any practitioner is equally capable, or incapable, as the original experimenter when it comes to getting the patient into the operating room.

One might also ask what happens when two studies give different values from ITT analysis. In the extreme case, one might suggest that if the same operation were recommended at a hospital in Newcastle-upon-Tyne as opposed to a battlefield in Iraq, the two ITT values would be different. So which is the appropriate one to attribute to that surgical procedure?

The ITT Controversy

Advocates of ITT see its principles as established and might dismiss a commonsense approach as naïve. They usually say that removing noncompliers introduces bias by destroying the original randomization. In this, they are confusing the process of randomization with the criteria for inclusion.

Case Study: Vitamin E Supplementation

A good case for the problems with ITT is a report on the value of antioxidant supplements. The abstract of the paper in question concluded that "there were no overall effects of ascorbic acid, vitamin E, or beta carotene on cardiovascular events among women at high risk for CVD." This conclusion—that there was no effect of supplementation—was based on an ITT analysis, but on the fourth page of the paper one can see the remarkable effect of not counting subjects who didn't comply: "Noncompliance led to a significant 13% reduction in the combined end point of CVD morbidity and mortality . . . with a 22% reduction in MI . . . , a 27% reduction in stroke . . . [, and] a 23% reduction in the combination of MI, stroke, or CVD death."

The media universally reported the conclusion from the abstract, namely, that there was no effect of vitamin E. This conclusion is correct if you think that you can measure the effect of vitamin E without taking the pill out of the bottle. (It's like the old joke about how you make a really dry martini: You don't remove the cap from the Vermouth bottle before pouring.) Does this mean that vitamin E is really of value? The data would certainly be accepted as valuable if the statistics were applied to a study of the value of, say, replacing barbecued pork with whole grain cereal. Certainly we can see that there is "no effect" when you tell a patient to take vitamin E, but that doesn't answer the question that most people are interested in: What are the effects when the patient *actually takes the vitamin?*

If you excluded people with diabetes from your study and only found out when the study started that one of the subjects actually had diabetes, like the tainted juries in courtroom dramas, you would be required to remove the individual anyway. You would not have included them if their diabetes came out in the voir dire, so you can't include them now. Of course, if you don't know whether a subject has actually complied, you are forced to include everybody, and that is what we have always done when there is no choice. That is not the issue here. The question is: What happens when you know who did and who didn't comply?

The problem is not easily resolved. Statistics is not axiomatic: There is nothing analogous to the zeroth law (the idea of thermal equilibrium on which thermodynamics rests). All statistics rests on interpretation and intuition. If this is not appreciated—if you do not go back to consideration of exactly what the question is that you are asking—it is easy to develop a dogmatic approach and insist on a particular methodology because it has become standard.

Assumption versus Consumption

Described in chapter 3 as the "shot heard 'round the world," Gary Foster's 2002 dietary study found that after one year, a low-carbohydrate diet was substantially better than a low-fat diet for markers of cardiovascular disease. When it came to weight loss, however, while the low-carbohydrate diet was better at six months, the two diets were "the same at one year." This, of course, was an effect of dwindling adherence in both the intervention and control groups, (although, in fact, the lipid markers were noticeably better on the low-carbohydrate group even at one year.)

A follow-up to the landmark one-year study, "Weight and Metabolic Outcomes after 2 Years on a Low-Carbohydrate Versus Low-Fat Diet,"[3] published in 2010, had a surprisingly limited impact. What went wrong? The first paper was revolutionary, and in the follow-up, the authors explicitly addressed the need for including a "comprehensive lifestyle modification program," because the original was criticized for simply giving the people on the Atkins diet a copy of the popular book. The criticism was addressed, and the conclusion was the same. The low-carbohydrate group had better outcomes for most CVD risk factors, although again, there was no difference in weight loss after two years. As stated in the conclusion: "Neither dietary fat nor carbohydrate intake influenced weight loss when combined with a comprehensive lifestyle intervention." This is, after all, still the party line and should have been well-received by establishment nutrition. That should have been a big win for the only-calories-count crowd. Why was there so little impact, and why is the paper so rarely cited?

It is likely that the zeitgeist has shifted since eight years ago. Strict scientific standards have suffered tremendous blows. The willingness to disregard the results of big expensive experiments and to ignore common sense is now much more widespread. Everybody knows—at this point—that in a big comparison trial, the low-carbohydrate diet will win in some way, and that it is likely that the authors will try to put a negative spin on things. As Elizabeth Nabel put it after the embarrassing Women's Health Initiative failure: "Nothing's changed." Low-fat is still the name of the game, a phrase in the USDA guidelines, and a component of the Healthy Hunger-Free Kids Act school lunch program[4] endorsed by Michelle Obama. Press releases on such government programs quote a progression of "suits" with maudlin expressions of optimism about how well what I call "Fruits 'n Vegetables" are doing in improving obesity. There are numerous disclaimers about good fats and bad fats, so that you can't really hold them to anything. However, since Foster's first study, numerous low-carbohydrate trials have showed it to be superior to any competition. Foster's 2010 study was, thus, not the challenge that the original was. It should, however, have been given some attention, at least because it was a follow-up to the landmark first paper. In my opinion, it deserved more attention primarily because it represented a new low in misleading science. The conclusion of the paper: "Neither dietary fat nor carbohydrate intake influenced weight loss."

I admit that I had not read Foster's paper carefully before making the pronouncement that it was not very good. I was even upbraided by a student for such a rush to judgment. I explained that that is what I do for a living. I explained that I usually don't have to spend a lot of time with a paper to get the general drift. I could easily see a couple of errors in methodology, which I describe below, but I was probably not totally convincing, so I went ahead and read the paper, which is quite a bit longer than usual. The main thing that I was looking for was information on the nutrients that were actually consumed, since it was their lack of effect that was the main point of the paper. The problem is that people feel that they can call anything that they want a low-carbohydrate diet, and of course, people really believe that being "assigned to a low-carbohydrate diet" is the same thing as consuming a low-carbohydrate diet. Frequently, when you look carefully at these studies, it turns out the diets were similar, so it is not surprising that the results are the same.

"Any Reasonably Intelligent High School Student"

In a diet experiment, the food consumed should be right up front, but in this case I couldn't find it at all. Foster's 2010 paper is quite long, with a tedious appendix on the lifestyle intervention, but I read the whole thing carefully. I really did. The data weren't there. I was going to write to the authors when I found out—I think through somebody's blog—that this paper had been covered in a story in the *Los Angeles Times*. As reported by Bob Kaplan:

> Of the 307 participants enrolled in the study, not one had their food intake recorded or analyzed by investigators. The authors did not monitor, chronicle or report any of the subjects' diets. No meals were administered by the authors; no meals were eaten in front of investigators. There were no self-reports, no questionnaires. . . . The lead authors, Gary Foster and James Hill, explained in separate e-mails that self-reported data are unreliable and therefore they didn't collect or analyze any.

I confess to feeling a bit shocked. How can you say "neither dietary fat nor carbohydrate intake influenced weight loss" if you haven't measured fat or carbohydrate? If you think that self-reported data are not good, then you can't make judgments about what was consumed. This would constitute a remarkable statement, since in fact the whole nutrition field runs on self-reported data. Are all the papers from the Harvard School of Public Health and all those epidemiology studies that rely on food records to be chucked out?

What would have happened if the authors had actually measured the relevant data—if they had asked what people eat, which, as Kaplan put it, is "the single most important question . . . that any reasonably intelligent high school student would ask." It's not just bad experimental design. It is a question of what is on their mind. Do they not realize that it is totally inappropriate to say that fat or carbohydrate are not important if they haven't measured them? They might be so biased that they don't see what is going on. In his first paper, Foster said in public, explicitly, that he set out to trash the Atkins diet. It's not a good way to do science. You are supposed to try to trash your own theory and show that it survives.

Beyond ITT: Fabricating Data

Foster's 2010 paper shows just how misleading ITT can be. Initially chastised for jumping to conclusions, I reread the paper carefully and one figure in particular caught my eye. The title: "Predicted Absolute Mean Change in Serum Triglycerides." Predicted? That sounds strange. What about the real data? The figure indicates changes in triglycerides for the three-, six-, twelve-, and twenty-four-month time periods.

Reduction in triglycerides is the hallmark of low-carbohydrate diets. Almost everybody on such a diet lowers their triglycerides (mine fell to half of the original value, a commonly reported outcome). In figure 16.1*A*, the difference in the levels of triglycerides between the two diets (shown by the double-headed arrow) was quite large at three or six months, the usual result. However, as the experiment continued, after twelve months, triglyceride values got closer and actually came together after twenty-four months.

This seemed strange, so I realized I had to find out where the word *predicted* came from, and that meant reading the methods section and going over the statistical analysis on how the data had been handled. In general, as mentioned before, you usually only read the methods section in detail if you think that it is a problem, or if a new method has been introduced, or if you want to repeat the author's experiment yourself. Large studies like this usually have a statistician, and they use standard methods whose details might or might not be understood by a nonstatistician (that's me) and most of the authors. They are usually accepted at face value and it is assumed that authors have adequately explained to the statistician what the question is that they want to address. As I kept plowing through the statistical section, I found it increasingly tedious and difficult to read until I hit this passage:

> The previously mentioned longitudinal models preclude the use of less robust approaches, such as fixed imputation methods

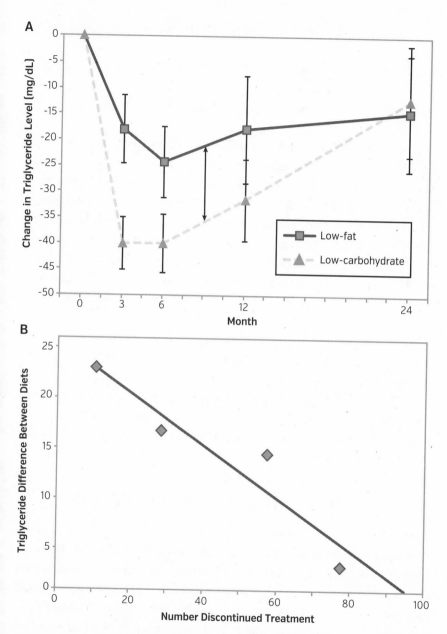

Figure 16.1. *A*, The double-headed arrow represents the difference between the change in triglycerides on the two indicated arms of the study. Figure redrawn from Foster et al. *B*, The distance shown by the arrow on the *y*-axis in part A (difference between the low-carbohydrate and low-fat groups) is shown as a function of the number of subjects who dropped out of the study.

(for example, last observation carried forward or the analysis of participants with complete data [that is, complete case analyses]). These alternative approaches assume that missing data are unrelated to previously observed outcomes or baseline covariates, including treatment (that is, missing completely at random).

Data "missing completely at random"? What's going on here? In a nutshell, this is another implementation of ITT. In the study, the authors used "data" from people who dropped out of the experiment. All they had to do was "assume that all participants who withdraw would follow first the maximum and then minimum patient trajectory of weight." The key words are *withdraw* and *assume*. This is really a step beyond ITT, where you would include, for example, the weight of people who showed up to be weighed but had not actually followed one or another diet. Here, nobody showed up. There are no data. A pattern of behavior is assumed and data are—let's face it—made up.

The world of nutrition puts big demands on irony and tongue-in-cheek, but the process in Foster's paper suggests that the results could, in theory, be fit to a model for a three-year study, or a ten-year study. As people dropped out you could "impute" the data. In some sense, you could do without any subjects at all. Nutrition experiments are expensive: Think of the money that could be saved if you didn't have to put anybody on a diet and you could make up all the data.

The Diet or the Lack of Compliance?

It is odd that ITT is controversial. In fact, it's odd that ITT exists at all. A reasonable way to deal with concern, however, that would satisfy everybody, is simply to publish both the ITT data and the data that include only the compliers, the so-called "per protocol" group—that is, the subjects that were actually in the experiment. This is what was done in the vitamin E study described in an earlier sidebar. It made the authors look bad, sure, but they did the right thing. Such data are missing from Foster's paper. Given the high attrition rate, one could guess that the decline in performance in both groups was due to including "data" from the large number of people who failed to complete the study. It turns out we can test this. The number of people who dropped out is in the paper. To find out whether the decline in performance is due to including the made-up data from the dropouts, we can plot the difference in triglycerides between the two groups (the double-headed arrow in figure 16.1*A*, for each time point, against the number of people who discontinued treatment.

Figure 16.1*B* gives you the answer. You can see a direct correlation between the number of dropouts and the group differences. The reason that "decreases in triglyceride levels were greater in the low-carbohydrate than in the low-fat group at 3 and 6 months but not at 12 or 24 months" was almost certainly because, with time, more and more people included in the data weren't on the low-carbohydrate diet, or any diet at all. ITT always makes the better diet look worse.

This serves as an example of a case where correlation strongly implies causality: The expectation from previous literature is that there will be a large difference in the level of triglycerides between the low-carbohydrate group and the low-fat group. (Decrease in triglycerides is virtually the definition of low-carbohydrate diets.) This expected difference was observed at the beginning of the trial, when the data were correlated with people actually taking part in the experiment. With time more people dropped out, so there were fewer people on either diet and, in turn, there was decreased difference between the groups—not being on a low-carbohydrate diet is, unsurprisingly, similar to not being on a low-fat diet. The take-home message is that ITT and imputing data will reduce the real effect of the intervention. In a diet experiment, the nature of the diet and compliance might be related—if the diet is unpalatable, people might not stay on it—but you have to show this. "Might" is not data. Along these lines, however, it is likely that the major reinforcer, the major reason people will stay on a diet, is that it works. In any case, one cannot assume that the two are linked without specifically testing the idea.

The Bottom Line

Intention-to-treat comes from the realization that in some experiments, you don't know who followed the protocol and who didn't. In a clinic, you might write a prescription and not know if it's been filled. In those cases, you have no choice but to include everybody's performance. However, the mechanical application of the idea in situations where you know who did or didn't comply is another misguided and dogmatic application of statistics. ITT usually makes the better diet look worse than it actually is. Awareness of whether this method has been used is important for evaluating a scientific publication.

CHAPTER 17

The Fiend
That Lies Like Truth

I pull in resolution and begin
To doubt th'equivocation of the fiend
That lies like truth.

— WILLIAM SHAKESPEARE, *Macbeth*

E rrors, inappropriate use of statistics, and misleading presentations are everywhere in the medical literature, as I've described in the previous chapters. Here I will summarize some of the specific problems we've covered and try to provide you with a guide to what to look for in the medical literature, and especially in the popular media.

Look for Visual Representations

You have a right to demand, and the author of a scientific paper has an obligation to provide, a clear explanation of what the results of their study really mean. A good test of whether or not the authors are holding up their end of the arrangement is the number and clarity of the figures. Visual presentation is almost always stronger than long tabulation of numbers. This principle is simultaneously so reasonable, and at the same time so widely violated, that Howard Wainer wrote a whole book, *Medical Illuminations*, arguing that scientific papers need more figures instead of the dense tables that make results hard to understand and force the reader to take the authors' conclusions at face value.[1]

Scientific publication is changing, and increasingly, as more and more journals become open access and available online, results of scientific studies will be universally available. An advantage to an open-access online journal is that there is no longer a limit on pages or number of figures. Nor is there an extra charge to the authors for the use of color in these figures. It is unknown how frequently authors take advantage of these opportunities, but the Golden Rule of Statistics remains the same: Let us see the data completely and clearly and in as many figures as it takes.

Science, but Not Rocket Science

"Eating breakfast reduces obesity" is not a principle from quantum electrodynamics. Most of us know whether or not eating breakfast makes us eat more or less during the day. Most of us also know that eating "good" anything is not good for losing weight—good might imply nutritious or tasty but usually means eating a lot. You don't need a physician, one who may have never studied nutrition, to tell you whether your perception is right or wrong. A degree in biochemistry is not required to understand the idea that adding sugar to your diet will increase your blood sugar—and the burden of proof is on anybody who wants to say that sugar is okay for people with diabetes. Anything is possible, but we start from what makes sense. Of course, there is technically sophisticated science and there are principles that require expertise to understand, but you should not automatically assume this is the case.

Be Suspicious of Self-Serving Descriptions

If a paper is about a diet that is described as "healthy," your appropriate answer should be, "that's for me to decide." The way the media tosses around the word *healthy* is bad enough, but in the context of a scientific paper it has to be considered an intellectual kiss of death. Nothing that you read after that can be taken at face value. If we knew what was healthy, we would not have an obesity epidemic and we would not need another paper to describe it.

Similarly, guidelines, data, or analyses that the authors describe as "evidence-based medicine" are likely to be deeply flawed. To use the court of law as an analogy: There must be a judge to decide admissibility of evidence. You can't pat yourself on the back and expect to be considered impartial. The courts have ruled that testimony by experts has to make sense, too. Credentials are not enough. As in the first principle, experts have to be able to explain data to the jury on the data's own merit. Be suspicious if the authors tell you how many other people agree with their position. Science does not run on "majority rules" or consensus.

Leaping Tall Buildings

As indicated in chapter 12, the new grand principle of doing science is *habeas corpus datorum*—in other words, let's see the body of the data. If the conclusion is counterintuitive and goes against previous work or common sense, then the data must be strong and clearly presented. Here's another way to put it: If you say you can jump over a chair, I can cut you a lot of slack and assume you're telling the truth. If you say you can jump over a building, however, I need to see you do it to be convinced. My daughter, at age nine, suggested an additional requirement. In a discussion of superheroes I pointed out that Superman used to be described as being "able to leap tall buildings in a single bound." She pointed out that if you try to leap tall buildings, you only get a single bound. You can't say your hundred-million-dollar, eight-year-long randomized controlled trial was not a fair test. The fat–cholesterol–heart hypothesis was sold as an absolute fact. None of the big clinical trials should have failed, but in the end, almost every single one did.

To return to the idea of "Let's see the body of the data": Show me what was done before you start running it through the computer. Statistics might be important, but in a diet experiment where one has to assume that even a well-defined population is heterogeneous, you want to understand how the individuals performed. The compelling work of Nuttall and Gannon,[2] for example, showing that diabetes can be improved even in the absence of weight loss, is increased in impact by the presentation of the individual performance. Not only is there general good response in reduction of blood glucose excursions, but all but two of the individual subjects benefited substantially, and all but one got at least somewhat better.

Understand Observational Studies

The usual warning offered by bloggers and others is that association does not imply causality, and that observational studies can only provide hypotheses for future testing. A more accurate description, as detailed in chapter 13, is that observational studies do not *necessarily* imply causality. Sometimes they do and sometimes they don't. The association between cigarette smoke and lung disease has a causal relation because the associations are very strong and because the underlying reason for making the measurement was based on basic physiology, including the understanding of nicotine as a toxin.

In this sense, observational studies test hypotheses rather than generating them. There are an infinite number of phenomena, but when you try to make a specific comparison between two, you usually have an idea in mind, conscious or otherwise. When a study tries to find an association between egg consumption and diabetes, it is testing the hypothesis that eggs are a factor in the generation of diabetes. It might not be sensible or based on sound scientific principles, but it's a hypothesis. If you do find a strong association with an unlikely hypothesis (this is the definition of intuition) then you have a new plausible hypothesis, and it must be further tested. It is important to question the hypothesis being tested in the first place, though. If the introduction section to the study says eggs have been associated with diabetes, you can at least check whether the reference is to an experimental study rather than a previous recommendation from some health agency.

Meta-Analysis and the End of Science

Doctors prefer a large study that is bad, to a small study that is good.

—Anonymous

While intention-to-treat is the most foolish activity plaguing modern medical literature, the meta-analysis is the most dangerous. In a meta-analysis you pool different studies to see if more information is available from the combination. As such it is inherently suspicious: If two studies have very different conditions, the results cannot sensibly be pooled. If, on the other hand, they are very similar, you have to ask why the results from the first study were not accepted. Finally, if the pooled studies give a different result than any of the individual studies, the authors are supposed

Group Statistics:
Bill Gates Walks into a Bar . . .

Everybody has their favorite example of how averages don't really tell you what you want to know, or how they are inappropriate for some situations. The reason most of these are funny is because they apply averages in cases where single events are important. One of my favorites, from the title of this sidebar: If Bill Gates walks into a bar, on average, everybody in the bar is a millionaire.

Technically speaking, averages start with the assumption that there is a kind of "true" value and that deviations are due to random error. If we could only control things well—if there were no wind resistance and each ball was absolutely uniform—all of the balls would always fall in the same place all the time. Any spread in values must be random rather than systematic. The familiar bell-shaped curve that illustrates the mean (average) value and deviations from the mean is referred to alternatively as the normal distribution or Gaussian distribution. Without going into details of statistics, the standard deviation, or SD, is supposed to give you a feel for how the real points deviate from the mean. From the SD, you can tell how reliable the data are. A low SD means that the mean value can be expected to be a reliable indication of what the actual data look like. A high SD, on the other hand, means that you can expect the data to be more spread out.

There are many examples. The textbooks cite the blitz in London in World War II when the V-1 "flying bombs" were distributed in a characteristic random pattern. ("Aiming" was presumed due to fixed launch sites and fixed fuel; deviations came from wind resistance and other random factors.) You can see a pretty good fit to the 3-D version of, in this case, the Poisson distribution.

On the other hand, Allied bombing of the German town of Aachen destroyed much of the city while leaving intact the famous cathedral where Charlemagne was crowned. The joke was that the cathedral was unharmed because that's what we were aiming at. It is generally assumed that what is good enough for bombing is good enough for social and biological science. But is it? Going from a large collection of individual points to two mathematical parameters (the mean and standard deviation), you obscure a good deal of information. A literally infinite number of different arrangements of points will give you the same mean and standard deviation.

Even more importantly, are you really sure that your data are uniform—that is, as the statisticians describe, that they come from the same population? Getting to the point: How are group statistics used in nutrition and medicine? The underlying principle is usually stated as the idea that "one size fits all." But is this a good idea? When we see a spread in weight loss on different diets, for example, is that due to minor individual variations (one subject always goes to the gym right after breakfast), or is it due to fundamental differences between people? For example, might there be two classes of people (e.g., insulin-sensitive and insulin-resistant)?

Nobody Loses an Average Amount of Weight

Use of averages depends on uniformity in the population. Yet in diet, we don't really believe that. Calling attention to all the people who eat more than you do and gain less weight than you do is considered an anecdotal observation. (The fact that you don't want to believe it adds some credibility.) There have been experiments, however. David Allison's group[3] studied a number of identical twins, putting them all on a weight-reduction diet for a month and measuring how much weight they lost. They calculated an energy deficit (differences between calories in and calories out) and compared that to the actual energy deficit (weight loss minus food intake).

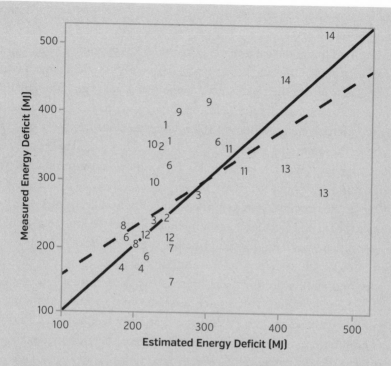

Figure 17.1. Relationship of estimated and measured energy deficit for fourteen twin pairs (same numbers). The dotted line is the regression of estimate on measured energy deficit, and the solid line represents identity (measured deficit = estimated). Subjects above the solid line (of identity) are absolutely less efficient than those below the line. Data from V. Rainer et al., "A Twin Study of Weight Loss and Metabolic Efficiency," *International Journal of Obesity and Related Metabolic Disorders* 25, no. 4 (2001): 533–537.

The pairs of twins in figure 17.1 were similar in their energy deficit, but there were major variations between twins. The study was carried out in a hospital but, given the possible random variations of twenty-eight people over the course of a month, this is pretty good evidence for what is popularly called "metabolic advantage" (people below the solid line) or maybe metabolic "disadvantage" (people above).

to point out what the original study did wrong (and the original authors are supposed to agree).

Simply adding more subjects is not considered a guarantee of reliability; however, papers in the medical literature frequently cite their large number of subjects as one of their strengths. If a meta-analysis is good for anything (which is questionable), it is for its originally intended role of evaluating small, underpowered studies with the hope that putting them together might reveal something you didn't originally see. It is a kind of "Hail Mary" last-ditch play. It was not intended for appropriately powered studies with a large number of subjects.

One of the benefits, conscious or unconscious, that keeps meta-analysis going is that it is perfect for current medical research. With meta-analysis, no experiment ever fails and no principle is ever disproved. Sugar causes heart attacks, cholesterol causes heart attacks, red meat causes heart attacks, and statins prevent heart attacks—it doesn't matter how many studies show no effect. One winner and you can do a meta-analysis. Just one more expensive trial and we'll show that saturated fat is bad. Plus you don't even have to explain what the previous researcher did wrong, as you might in a real experiment.

The idea that simply adding more subjects will improve reliability is not reasonable. Most of us think that if a phenomenon has large variability, then mixing studies will reduce predictability although it might sharpen statistical significance. And again, in science it is expected that if your results contradict previous experiments, you will provide evidence as to the cause of the differences. What did previous investigators do wrong? Do those investigators now agree that you've improved things? Probably not, especially if you don't ask them.

Be Suspicious of Grand Principles

"Randomized controlled trials are the gold standard." "Metabolic ward studies are the gold standard." "Observational studies are only good for generating hypotheses." Such grand principles do not play a part in the physical sciences, where the method that we choose depends on the question that we want to answer. You do not need to carry out a long-term trial to see if a treatment is appropriate for an acute condition. You do not need

Saturated Fatty Acids, Carbohydrates, and Meta-Analysis

A number of important meta-analyses have examined the effect of saturated fatty acids on cardiovascular risk. They all show a very small benefit if the saturated fatty acids are replaced with carbohydrate. Examination of the data, however, reveals that almost all of the included studies failed to show any significant effect of replacing saturated fat, and yet the authors came up with an answer. How is this possible? It is the consequence of group-think. If everybody—the editors, the reviewers, and ultimately the reader—assumes that meta-analysis is an acceptable method, then peer review will be meaningless.

a randomized controlled study to find out whether penicillin is effective for treating gram-positive infections. Penicillin is a drug and you might have to do a randomized controlled trial to determine safety, but at the efficacy end, if the results are clear-cut, only a small number of tests are necessary. How many? It depends on how many people recover spontaneously. A statistician can figure this out for you if you ask the question appropriately.

The idea of the randomized controlled trial as a gold standard has really never recovered from Smith and Pell's landmark paper, "Parachute Use to Prevent Death and Major Trauma Related to Gravitational Challenge: Systematic Review of Randomised Controlled Trials."[4] In the paper, Smith and Pell concluded that "the effectiveness of parachutes has not been subjected to rigorous evaluation by using randomised controlled trials."

Described as both funny and profound, the paper included all the relevant information, making fun of the excessive statistical detail in the literature: "We chose the Mantel-Haenszel test to assess heterogeneity, and sensitivity and subgroup analyses and fixed effects weighted regression techniques to explore causes of heterogeneity. We selected a funnel plot to assess publication bias visually and Egger's and Begg's tests to test it quantitatively."

Smith and Pell pointed out that there were only two solutions to the problem of a lack of randomized controlled trials: "The first is that we accept that, under *exceptional* circumstances, *common sense* might be applied when considering the potential risks and benefits of interventions. The second is that we continue our quest for the holy grail of exclusively evidence-based interventions and preclude parachute use outside the context of a properly conducted trial." (Emphasis added)

In the end, the authors suggested that "those who advocate evidence-based medicine and criticise use of interventions that lack an evidence base . . . demonstrate their commitment by volunteering for a double blind, randomised, placebo controlled, crossover trial."

The bottom line is that science has to make sense and does not depend on arbitrary rules. Smith and Pell made fun of how often authors attempt to snow us. There really are statistical tests with those names, but science is not about fixed rules and accounting. It is about understanding each experiment and knowing the question to be asked.

The faults that plague the medical literature have made it a minefield for readers, and more often than not, readers will not be happy with the latest study showing that processed food or one or another of the usual suspects will kill you. Armed with a few principles, you can understand what is explicitly wrong with these studies that so strongly violate common sense. Failure to show individual data; the use of questionable practices, such as intention-to-treat and meta-analyses; and, most of all, failure to actually apply common sense, are the things to look for. It will be hard to accept that the Harvard School of Public Health, all the best and the brightest, could be making elementary mistakes, but the proof and precedents are there.

PART 5

The Second Low-Carbohydrate Revolution

CHAPTER 18

Nutrition in Crisis

"More work needs to be done" is the standard conclusion of weak dietary studies or those that got the "wrong answer." As in any biological science, what we know is much less than what we don't know. When it comes to moving forward on the low-carbohydrate argument, however, no more work needs to be done: Switching from your current diet to a low-carbohydrate or ketogenic diet is usually the healthiest change you can make. We know this because it has been put to the test. After being subjected to forty years of persistent criticism—some rigorous, some preposterous and outlandish, some virulent—carbohydrate restriction has proven to be the most effective way to lose weight and the first line of treatment for diabetes.

Yet for forty years, the medical and nutritional establishment have pulled out all the stops in a compulsive effort to find something medically wrong with low-carbohydrate diets. They've come up with nothing at all. In head-to-head comparisons, regardless of the length of the trials, low-carbohydrate almost always wins. At the same time, we have forty years of multicenter, multimillion-dollar trials that fail to show any risk from total fat or saturated fat or dietary cholesterol. We need to face—and capitalize on—the scientific data that stand clearly before us before any more work needs to be done.

For the individual dieter, we have found the optimal strategy. It's not a magic bullet, and it's not something that works the same for everybody, but it's the best we have. The challenge now is to work out a plan to implement the low-carbohydrate strategy. The crisis in nutrition is that you might be on your own. Your physician or health provider is not guaranteed to be on your side and might, in fact, be trying to dissuade you from the best course of action. If you're lucky, and your provider is reasonable, you might be able to teach them. A physician, in particular, might have no training at all in nutrition, and the practice of analyzing original research critically is unlikely to be part of their daily activity, so you can point them to relevant literature. *Nutrition in Crisis* would be a good start.

Twilight of the Lipophobes

So how close are we to good science and good guidance on nutrition? I spoke at the LEO Conference, held in Gothenburg, Sweden, which celebrates nonconformity in science. The 2008 meeting honored Uffe Ravnskov, the arch cholesterol skeptic.[1] Quoting Max Planck, speakers before me suggested that if you really wanted to introduce a new idea in science, you had to wait for the old generation to die out. When I spoke,[2] I suggested that since I was in that generation, we might want to do it a little sooner.

How far do we have to go? As in any highly contentious field, the answer you get depends on whom you ask. While low-fat still hangs over everything, there are now numerous disclaimers: "Only saturated fat is a risk" or maybe it's only a problem if "you replace polyunsaturated fat with saturated fat." The large, expensive, randomized controlled trials that successfully showed no effect of dietary total saturated fat or cholesterol are still assumed to have never taken place—and although the case for low-carbohydrate and its benefits is established, the best that can be done according to many is to claim that "it is not any better" than low-fat diets, despite the fact that low-fat never wins, and only ever draws. Attacking sugar is considered a first step—presumably because sugar is an easy target. Whether the second step, if there really is one, is a more comprehensive meaningful low-carbohydrate recommendation, is never stated. It is a political strategy that involves fundamental disdain for the audience, and one that is almost guaranteed to backfire.

Things are progressing, yes. Many researchers and organizations, while admitting no wrongdoing, are slowly giving in to low-carbohydrate. Yet there is simultaneously unrestrained backlash, which has taken a very ugly turn toward personal and professional attacks on low-carbohydrate researchers and journalists.

Quashing Dissent around the World

Coincidentally, it was in Sweden that the medical establishment revealed its resistance to criticism and to new ideas. Dr. Annika Dahlqvist lives in

Njurunda, Sundsvall. She described on her blog[3] how she discovered that a low-carbohydrate diet would help in her own battle with obesity and various health problems that included enteritis (irritable bowel syndrome, or IBS), gastritis, fibromyalgia, chronic fatigue syndrome, insomnia, and snoring. Recommending low-carbohydrate diets for her patients and publicly advertising her ideas drew a certain amount of media attention, leading to a run-in with the authorities. In November 2006 she lost her job at Njurunda Medical Center. She was ultimately exonerated in January 2008, when the National Board of Health and Welfare found that a low-carbohydrate diet was "consistent with good clinical practice." This was the likely prelude to the announcement in 2013 that the Swedish Agency for Health Technology Assessment, which is charged with assessing national health care treatment, endorsed low-carbohydrate diets for weight loss. While their statements were far from enthusiastic, it was one of a number of events that indicated the fall of the low-fat paradigm and the no-holds-barred backlash of nutritional medicine.

The most bizarre case, which was resolved as I was finishing this book, occurred in Australia. An orthopedic surgeon, Dr. Gary Fettke, had become the target of the Australian Health Practitioner Regulation Agency (AHPRA) after he publically discussed the benefits of a low-carb diet. In a letter dated November 1, 2016, the AHPRA told Fettke, "There is nothing associated with your medical training or education that makes you an expert or authority in the field of nutrition, diabetes or cancer."[4] The ensuing persecution was remarkably unprofessional and ugly, and it wasn't until nearly two years later that the AHPRA exonerated Fettke and offered a belated and inadequate apology. The training of any physician in nutrition is, in my view, problematic, but it has been rightly pointed out, in response to the original letter, that Fettke received the same training as other doctors.

The letter continued: "Even if, in the future, your views on the benefits of the [low-carb, high-fat] LCHF lifestyle become the accepted best medical practice, this does not change the fundamental fact that you are not suitably trained or educated as a medical practitioner to be providing advice or recommendations on this topic as a medical practitioner." In short, even if the AHPRA recognized the truth, they would not defend Fettke's right to say it. As many noted at the time, Dr. Fettke is in fact trained to remove the limbs of those whose diabetes has reached a critical point, despite the AHPRA's attempts to diminish his credentials. This lack of due process and common decency speaks to the need for some kind of regulation. The issue hasn't receive significant coverage in traditional media, which have kept it relatively invisible, but the recent turn of events may bring out just how bad things are. The fallout from this scandal is just being uncovered, and Marika Sboros's blog, foodmed.net, is a likely source for the unfolding story. Her recent blog post titled "Fettke: Cover-Up Grows After Case Against Him Collapses?" is both gripping and intensely distressing.

Stateside, a North Carolina blogger named Steve Cooksey was enjoined from recommending a low-carbohydrate diet for diabetes by the North Carolina Board of Dietetics/Nutrition. After a near-death experience from his own diabetes, and after experiencing the benefits of carbohydrate restriction, he felt it might be good to share the information with others, with due disclaimers about not offering medical advice. That was too much for the professional nutritionists who somehow have gotten the state legislature to designate them as sole purveyors of nutritional advice. Enlisting the aid of the Institute for Justice, Cooksey won a First Amendment lawsuit and the North Carolina board realized that it could not tell American citizens what they could and could not say. The board changed its guidelines, but the fury of a nutritionist spurned is great—and even worse down under.

The Dietitians Association of Australia (DAA) registers dietitians and essentially controls whether they can do their jobs in hospitals, universities, or private practice. In 2015, the DAA expelled Jennifer Elliott, a dietitian with thirty years' experience and a highly regarded book for patients. She had also published a peer-reviewed critique of the diet–heart hypothesis, which likely contributed to the DAA action. The complaint from a DAA-registered dietitian was that Elliott's recommendation of low-carbohydrate diets for her patients with type 2 diabetes was not "evidence-based." The DAA upheld the complaint. In my personal communication with Claire Hewat, head of the DAA, however, she claimed that the cause of dismissal had not been the recommendations of low-carbohydrate diet but something else that could not be revealed because it was confidential. The power of low-carbohydrate diets to provoke hostile behavior remains fascinating if incomprehensible. In a blog post on the subject, I made an analogy to the Protestant Reformation, although unlike

The Tim Noakes Case

*It is troublesome to hear that Tim is being attacked
so strongly for what seems to be a trivial matter,
when there are plenty of real problems in health
care and our world more broadly.*
—WALTER WILLETT[5]

Most bizarre for its virulence remains the determination with
which the Health Professionals Council of South Africa
(HPSCA) tried to maintain control by attacking Tim Noakes.
A retired physician and widely admired sports expert, and only a
relatively recent spokesman for carbohydrate restriction, Noakes
answered a comment on Twitter that suggested a newborn
could be weaned to a low-carbohydrate diet, not particularly
different from the recommendations of Australian authorities.
Yes, this is about a single tweet, which wasn't even taken into
account by the individual who'd asked the question in first place.
A nutritionist was insulted by the affair and brought the case
to the HPSCA. The question become whether Noakes's tweet
constituted medical advice—the primary affirmative argument
being that because he was a medical doctor, anything Noakes
said could be considered advice. This is just as ridiculous as the
folk myth that a black belt in karate has to register his hands at
local police stations as lethal weapons.

The HPSCA came down hard on Noakes but, after two
years of trial, he was exonerated. The HPCSA's own committee
found that no harm derived from the tweet, and that his advice
was "evidence-based" and within normal standards. HPSCA
was able to establish a warning for other medical professionals, since as Noakes explained, "It's been very, very demanding
on us and on our lives and financially it's been huge." Noakes
asked, further, "Did they ever consider the consequences for my

wife and myself and our family?" Indicating that it did not, the HPSCA immediately appealed the decision of its own committee. While the decision of the new body was supposed to be produced with all deliberate speed, innate pettiness presumably caused them to drag it out for months. Noakes was finally exonerated. Besides being a person of stature in sports medicine, he is a charming, friendly person—I met him at a landmark conference at Ohio State University just as the final edits on this book were prepared.

Luther, Jennifer Elliott was not particularly rebellious and was not trying to reform anything except her patients' dietary habits. The DAA functions, after all, as a professional dietitians' organization and should, as in *Macbeth*, against the murder shut the door, not bear the knife itself. There was some press coverage but little public awareness or professional outcry over the lack of natural justice and common decency.

Dissent will not be tolerated. When Nina Teicholz, author of *The Big Fat Surprise*, published a critical analysis in the *BMJ* describing excesses of the expert report by the HHS-USDA Dietary Guidelines Advisory Committee (DGAC)—notably that it did not even discuss low-carbohydrate diets—Michael Jacobson, the obsessive and humorless leader of the Center for Science in the Public Interest (CSPI, a largely vegetarian watchdog group), initiated a petition to have the paper retracted because it was "so riddled with errors." The alleged errors turned out to be less about Teicholz's scientific conclusions than about who used what database as evidence. From Jacobson's petition: "Teicholz states that 'in the NEL systematic review on saturated fats from 2010 . . . fewer than 12 small trials are cited, and none supports the hypothesis that saturated fats cause heart disease. . . .' Correction: It is incorrect to state that none of the trials cited in the 2010 NEL review supports the hypothesis."

The paper was not retracted, presumably because no scientific issue was raised and Teicholz's critique was judged "within the realm of scientific debate." A revealing bit of information was exposed along the way, however: Frank Hu of Harvard School of Public Health, lead author of the DGAC review of saturated fats, personally sent out multiple emails to colleagues, putting together a posse of more than 150 people, including many graduate students, who ultimately signed the CSPI petition. The petition remains problematic in that it did not represent an assembly of people who had expressed concern, but rather an assortment of people who were contacted by Dr. Hu with an unsolicited request to sign the petition.

The Big Picture

The extent to which repressive behavior actually reduces research on or acceptance of dietary carbohydrate restriction is unknown. However, the hostile, personal attacks—generally uncharacteristic of scientific behavior—represent desperation. If they could actually deal with the issue on a scientific basis, they wouldn't have to behave like this. It is likely, however, that the aggression is a response to seeing people, including their patients, find out the answer for themselves.

The studies from Volek's lab are particularly compelling, but in fact, almost every comparison in the scientific literature shows that low-carbohydrate diets are more effective for weight loss and most other metabolic disturbances. The rationale is that dietary carbohydrate is the major stimulus for secretion of the anabolic hormone insulin. Chapter 9 explained how it is possible to lose more weight, calorie for calorie, on a low-carbohydrate diet: The bottom line is that insulin slows the breakdown (lipolysis) of fat, and if you consume another meal before the system has had a chance to deal with stored fat, it will accumulate. Also, on a low-carbohydrate diet, your appetite goes down—satiety is increased, so most people find it easier to adhere to a carbohydrate-restricted diet than to any other.

The real win for low-carbohydrate diets is personal: It changes your interaction with food. For people with a weight problem, every meal is a battle. Every time you sit down at the table you're trying to make sure you don't cross some line of calories, fat, or whatever other metric you're keeping an eye on. If you make a substantial cut in the amount of carbohydrates that you eat, even if you are not overly precise, even if you spend a couple of days at the conference buffet, you are unlikely to gain any weight. You lose a substantial part of your obsession with and anxiety about food.

It is reassuring, too, to know that we don't have a biological need for carbohydrate and that the opposite of lowering fat intake is not eating all the fat in sight. It might well be true, as critics of low-carbohydrate diet say, that the recommended low-carbohydrate strategy includes assurances that "you can eat all the fat that you want," but the emphasis is on "want." Fat is filling. How much do you want? It is important to stress that the low-fat idea was not originally instituted to deal with obesity but rather to prevent heart disease (which it didn't) and it always had a moralistic overtone. It was somebody's idea of what we should have been eating during the millennia in which haute cuisine evolved and people perfected sausages and other food in ethnic cuisines. The low-fat idea was the work of Puritans. It gave rise to the obesity epidemic, and the fact that many people did not get fat is only a testament to the adaptability of humans in dealing with all kinds of food.

The real impact of low-carbohydrate and ketogenic diets is the tie to biologic mechanism and the generality of control of metabolism by insulin and associated hormones. From a scientific standpoint, the main ideas are established, and all that remains is political and social acceptance. As this acceptance sets in, our understanding of metabolic control mechanisms might unlock new and exciting possibilities.

CHAPTER 19

Cancer

A New Frontier for Low-Carbohydrate

I t was in July 2012 that I realized we'd won. It was now clear that we had a consistent set of scientific ideas supporting the central role of insulin signaling in basic biochemistry. We could see a continuum with the effectiveness of dietary carbohydrate restriction for obesity, diabetes, and general health. The practical considerations—how much to eat of this, how much to eat of that—hadn't yet been fully resolved, but we had the kernel of a scientific principle. In fact, it was not so much that we had the answer as that we had the right question. We were, at last, looking at diet, metabolism, and disease as a single entity. We were asking whether pathologic changes could be precisely traced back to disease, and that meant focusing on the downstream effects of high-carbohydrate intake. In science, the question is frequently more important than the answer. If you know what to look for, you are more likely to find it. Of course it wasn't originally about winning, or even fighting. When my colleagues and I got into this about ten years earlier, coming from a background of basic biochemistry, we hadn't anticipated that it would be such a battle, that there would be so much resistance to what we thought was normal scientific practice. Surprisingly, it was cancer studies that made clear how it all fit together, and seemed to signal the success of all our work.

We generally recognize cancer as a genetic disease—not necessarily inherited, but a disease associated with genetic mutations. A great deal of research has gone into identifying the mutations and where the products of the mutant genes fit in. While this has given rise to much valuable information, it has been impossible to identify a single mechanism for cancer. Numerous mutations have been identified but finding a common thread has rarely been possible—and the information we do have has led to only a small number strategies, pharmaceutical or otherwise, for treatment or prevention.

The focus of cancer research, however, has recently begun to turn back to earlier studies on the relation of energy metabolism to the cancerous state. With this shift in focus, researchers have paid greater attention to the Warburg effect, the observation that many tumors rely on glycolysis—the anaerobic processing of glucose to pyruvic acid described in chapter 5. The re-appreciation of energy metabolism has had wide-ranging consequence. This is not to say that the genetic mutation theory has somehow been replaced by a metabolic theory. In fact, it is usually impossible to separate genetic and metabolic effects. Metabolism runs on enzymes, which are proteins, and proteins are primarily controlled by their synthesis, the gene products. In other words, although you could consider DNA to be a blueprint, that blueprint is not simply copied and sent out to the factory. Rather, we keep going back to the blueprint, and the workers vote on whether the body will work on one or another part of the blueprint, and choose what to do with each piece created. This slightly strained analogy means that the total state of the cell, its energy profile and cell constituents, will determine which proteins stipulated by the genome will be expressed and the extent to which they will be active. The focus on metabolism was the thread that brought us back to nutrition and the control of energy production and utilization. There suddenly seemed to be better appreciation of the need for a nutritional approach. I felt that we had reached some kind of turning point.

The locale was a conference in Washington, DC, called "Metabolism, Diet and Disease." It might have been better billed as "Metabolism, Drugs and Cancers," at least based on the first day, but there was a surprising thread in the various talks—surprising to me, at least—about the very strong association between obesity and risk of cancer. Less surprising to me, because of the numerous studies I'd read, were the presentations about the effect of total dietary calorie restriction, the apparent basis for the connection between obesity and cancer: Reducing calories has been shown to reliably increase longevity and to control cancer in animals. An additional element of the conversation was the hormone insulin, which had popped up as a major player in various experiments on cancer. Then there was the identification of downstream signaling elements—the compounds and proteins that transmit the information about cell stimulation to the interior of the cell. These were important results, and again, they frequently pointed to the components of insulin pathways and even to an association between cancer and diabetes. This last point was not entirely new to me: Outstanding experiments had indicated the critical role of insulin, and I always wondered why the connection to dietary carbohydrate hadn't been made. In any case, the second day of the conference included presentations on dietary carbohydrate restriction, and although he was not listed on the organizing committee, Gary Taubes had helped set up the event and deserves credit for bringing together cancer people and low-carbohydrate people.

My colleague Dr. Eugene Fine presented a poster at the Washington conference. Many conferences have poster sessions: Presenters pin posters, typically four by six feet, to easels, and attendees at the conference can then discuss the subject matter with the presenter. Posters don't always have a big impact, so we were grateful to Gary Taubes for making Eugene's poster known to the main speakers. The paper on which the poster was based, now published in the journal *Nutrition*,[1] describes a small study conducted with ten seriously ill cancer patients. The study had the modest goal of showing that a ketogenic diet was a safe and feasible regimen, and in fact, the patients did well. Six of the ten stabilized or went into partial remission. By itself, this study would be considered only a small step forward, but in fact, it was key in tying together the fields of carbohydrate restriction and cell signaling in the context of normal and cancer cells. The experiment was difficult to do: The patients had to have refused or failed chemotherapy and exhausted all the traditional regimens. Yet it was incredibly significant. Given what we know about insulin and low-carbohydrate diets, the experiment should have been done twenty years ago. These two lines of thought simply had to be brought together.

In hindsight, it seems that workers in carbohydrate restriction should have paid more attention to downstream cell signaling. We thought that the role of insulin in system biochemistry made it clear that carbohydrate restriction was built on a solid foundation. The resistance to the idea seemed incomprehensible and parochial, but this conference made it obvious that more was needed to form a consistent biological story. It became clear that there was a conceptual barrier to acceptance of carbohydrate restriction beyond the traditional resistance to anything associated with the Atkins diet. There were additional factors. There was a mind-set that prevented adequate synthesis of all the information.

Targeting Cancer through Insulin Inhibition

When approaching cancer, much of the valuable work in cell biology tended to downplay the biochemistry at the upstream-stimulus level—namely, what you eat and its immediate biologic consequences. The major goal had been to characterize the individual components in the inner working of the cell and to search for those components that were specifically malfunctioning in pathological states. These agents—primarily proteins and the associated genes from which they were expressed—could then be targeted with drugs, either directly or indirectly at the genomic level. With the important observation that calorie restriction could ameliorate or prevent cancer, a link with obesity was established, and in some way excess calories became interchangeable with weight gain. The obesity–cancer link became a serial link and it was assumed—as it is frequently assumed in nutrition— that preventing obesity was part of preventing associated pathologies. As a result of this framing, successes of carbohydrate restriction in improving cardiovascular risk factors, for example, have frequently been dismissed as due to the attendant weight loss. This, despite the evidence that the improvements in risk factors or other outcomes persist even in the absence of weight loss, or even when benefits were demonstrated in eucaloric trials.

The rationale of the research, then, was that calorie restriction—the recognized approach to obesity—would point to those intracellular components that could be targeted for drug development. In many cases this was a conceptual error. In nutrition it is likely that the doctrine of "a calorie is a calorie" is the single greatest impediment to understanding. Otherwise sophisticated and informative experiments were compromised by the identification of obesity with excess calories, and the failure to look beyond this effect—by the failure to ask how the separate nutrients, carbohydrate, fat, and protein, individually affect cellular metabolism, and how these effects interact (there is, after all, no calorie receptor). Similarly, as I mentioned above, I and other workers in carbohydrate restriction failed to see how important it was to look at downstream cellular signaling.

Fine's study treated ten seriously ill cancer patients with low-carbohydrate ketogenic diets and showed that it was a safe and feasible regimen for such patients. The rationale followed from the fact that rapidly growing tumors have a requirement for glucose, but simply reducing carbohydrates to give the host an advantage was unlikely to be effective because blood glucose is regulated to stay fairly constant and the cancers are good at getting whatever glucose is there. Tumors overexpress GLUT1 protein, the non-insulin-dependent glucose receptors. The odds were therefore strongly stacked against us when it came to effectively depriving the cancer of glucose. The question was whether ketone bodies, the specific consequence of very low-carbohydrate intake, might themselves exert control over the cancer cells.

Ketosis, the state associated with very low-energy or very low-carbohydrate intake, held some promise. Fine hypothesized that if we think of cancer in terms of genetics, we could think of cancer cells as having evolved throughout the life of the individual, an individual whose systemic environment, in a modern setting, would be unlikely to experience any significant level of ketosis—and that would therefore be unlikely to provide any selective pressure for the adaptation to use of ketone bodies as a fuel source. The host, on the other hand, was well adapted to this substrate: It is unlikely that our ancestors regularly had three square meals a day. Some fraction of cancer lines, then, might not deal well with a ketotic environment.

In the experiment it turned out that those patients who became stable or showed partial remission had the highest level of ketone bodies. Figure 19.1*A* shows individual time points with different symbols for each patient. As expected, there was a correlation between ketone bodies and insulin levels.

Although this was a small sample, figure 19.1*B* shows that while some of the patients had progressive disease, some became stable or showed partial remission. The level of ketone bodies was the best predictor of this outcome. Figure 19.1*C* shows, on the other hand, that improvements did not depend on calories or weight loss. Patients who demonstrated stable disease or partial remission had a threefold higher average ketotic response compared to those with continued progressive disease. However, both groups showed similar calorie deficits, or, as shown, degree of weight

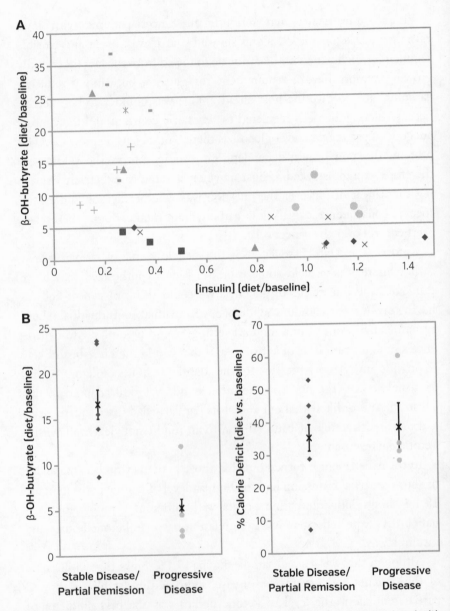

Figure 19.1. *A*, Ketonemia versus insulinemia: The lowest insulinemia correlated with the highest ketonemia levels. Different symbols represent values for each patient. *B*, Ketosis versus disease progression: Patients who demonstrated stable disease or partial remission had much greater ketotic response compared to those with progressive disease. *C*, Calorie deficit versus outcome: The stable disease/partial remission and progressive disease groups showed no difference in calorie reduction.

loss—suggesting that the well-established benefits in caloric restriction reflect an underlying mechanism beyond the energy itself.

Nailing the Link

A small study in advanced cancer patients might be considered only a minor step forward, but in fact it ties into a vast area of research on the downstream signaling in both cancer and normal cells—that is, the changes in the cell following stimulation by an external food or hormones. Of particular interest is the well-known effect of calorie restriction. It was widely understood that dietary calorie restriction would have a therapeutic effect on animals with cancer, and in addition, that reducing calories was the only way to prolong life in animals. Studies following this idea showed that it was an insulin pathway that was involved. Eugene Fine's study nailed the link for us. It is an encouraging situation, because if this is the worst of times in nutrition, it is also the golden age of biology. Bringing all of the science to bear on the problem has great promise indeed.

–CHAPTER 20–

The Future of Nutrition

The low-carbohydrate revolution of 2002 was precipitated by the popular exposés on the low-fat-diet–heart hypothesis and its consistent failure to find support in large clinical trials. The well-armed forces mustered by the diet–heart hypothesis fared poorly in the early confrontations with the actual experimental evidence. It was a case of failure to accept failure, even as authorities tried to generalize the proposed harm of dietary fat to obesity and diabetes. Scientific developments, however, have continued to reinforce the idea that control of metabolism by insulin and other hormones is the key factor in weight loss, diabetes, metabolic syndrome, and—now—perhaps even cancer. Classic, well-controlled experiments have nailed the idea: Carbohydrate restriction is the best therapy for all of the features of metabolic syndrome and the default treatment for diabetes, consistent with its nature as a disease of carbohydrate intolerance.

At the same time, underwhelming tests of the diet–heart hypothesis continue to be conducted, despite the base of evidence to the contrary. Support comes from meta-analyses and epidemiological statistical juggling, whose minimal positive outcomes—again, an odds ratio of 1.5 seems even worse if described as 60:40—are just as damning as the well-documented failures. Bias against publishing studies of low-carbohydrate diets seems as strong as ever. A low-carbohydrate paper submitted to the *New England Journal of Medicine*, the *BMJ*, or other major journals will be treated with superficial politeness if you're lucky, or—more likely—palpable disdain.

For scientists and consumers alike, the situation has become more confusing, more ambiguous. A major factor appears to be a near disintegration of standards. Epidemiologic studies trying to show the risks in saturated fat (good fats–bad fats), in red meat, in sugar (good carbs–bad carbs) continue to proliferate. In the absence of critical peer review, they are accepted for publication, and their conclusions are presented at face value in the media, and notably in the online medical publications from which physicians receive much of their information. The same journals and popular medical sites publish papers describing how bad the obesity epidemic is, and directly, or by implication, blame the patient. Ironically these journals also publish articles lamenting the very breakdown in standards in the medical literature to which they are the primary contributors.[1]

The effects of carbohydrate per se are generally ignored. If they are mentioned at all, it is always to point out the dangers of "refined" carbohydrate. Wild, exaggerated dangers are attributed to sugar and high-fructose corn syrup, which are misguidedly separated from carbohydrates at large, and the lipophobes seem to have maintained control of the market: Low-fat versions of nearly every product, even "half and half," are pushed in the supermarkets. Yet, at the same time, there is a sense that it is all over. The accumulating failures of low-fat and the popular books and articles exposing those failures are finally taking their toll. The publication in 2014 of Nina Teicholz's *The Big Fat Surprise* might well be the second low-carbohydrate revolution's *Common Sense*, but whatever ultimately deals the death blow, it is clear that the nutritional establishment has cracked. Squabbling among the proponents of low-fat is a sure sign.

What's Next?

It is, perhaps, the end of the beginning.

—WINSTON CHURCHILL

It is clear that low-fat is dead. Burying it seems like a good idea. Continual failures of large trials, in combination with the success of alternative approaches, especially control of metabolism through the glucose–insulin axis, makes a new method of thinking inevitable.

Surprisingly, the key scientific focus of the second low-carbohydrate revolution might be cancer. It has long been recognized that total caloric restriction, at least in animals, is of benefit in slowing progression of disease and extending life. This has led to the questionable paradigm of identifying calories with obesity and identifying obesity, in turn, as a stimulus for pathological effects. One problem is that calorie restriction, as implemented, generally involves intentional or de facto reduction in carbohydrate. Moreover, calorie restriction is too broad a term to provide much insight on mechanism, whereas we have substantial understanding of the biochemical effects of individual macronutrients, and especially the role of insulin.

Research in carbohydrate restriction has probably underestimated the importance and value of detailed downstream stimulus–response coupling in cells, while cell biology has paid insufficient attention to the nature of upstream signaling—the effect of diet. It is not calories but carbohydrate that stimulates insulin release, and obesity is largely a response, not a stimulus. Ketone bodies, too, are vital to our evolving understanding. Originally considered primarily a marker for fat breakdown, ketone bodies are now understood to be a more global cell signal. The possibility of cancer treatment based on the theory that tumors might be more poorly adapted to use ketone bodies as an energy source because of their evolution during the life span of the individual is one specific approach tested in Eugene Fine's small pilot study.[2]

More generally, the use of carbohydrate restriction as a cancer therapy might be *the* important battleground in the search for effective dietary treatment and prevention. The new scientific paradigm might also be better received in the area of oncology due to the failures of other methods to contain the disease. With regard to obesity, diabetes, and metabolic diseases, it may be necessary to clear out the backlog of biased, unscientific, and statistically flawed studies that have so far impeded progress. New standards will have to be implemented to improve the future literature. Scientific truth is its own justification, but in this case, relief of human suffering is what is truly important to society at large. Progress may be slow but the crisis is real and the stakes are high.

ACKNOWLEDGMENTS

Two people, Monika Hendry and Paula Nedved, have made this book possible. Their continual encouragement, their probing questions, and their excellent proofreading abilities kept the book alive through periods during which there were many doubts and discouragements. I am also grateful to Professor Wendy Pogozelski for her help with chapter 2 and for her enthusiasm about the final product.

Insofar as this book is scientifically accurate it is due to my early influences, particularly Thomas C. Detwiler, and later interactions with my colleagues, Doctors Eugene J. Fine, Frederick Sacks, Jeff S. Volek, Eric C. Westman, Jay Wortman, Steve Phinney, Ann Childers, and many others who have for so long served as loyal opposition to the medical and nutritional monarchy.

Thanks also to members of the Nutrition and Metabolism Society and Facebook friends, as well as the greater social circle, Gary Taubes, Nina Teicholz, Carole Friend, Judy Barnes Baker, and especially the pseudonymous Amanda B. Wreckondwith, who have provided continuous encouragement and endured a certain degree of curmudgeonly behavior. I am grateful to the State University of New York Downstate Medical Center, which has given me the freedom to work and think outside the box.

NOTES

Introduction

1. W. Pogozelski, N. Arpaia, and S. Priore, "The Metabolic Effects of Low-Carbohydrate Diets and Incorporation into a Biochemistry Course," *Biochemistry and Molecular Biology Education* 33 (2005): 91–100; R. D. Feinman and M. Makowske, "Metabolic Syndrome and Low-Carbohydrate Ketogenic Diets in the Medical School Biochemistry Curriculum," *Metabolic Syndrome and Related Disorders* 1 (2003): 189–98; M. Makowske and R. D. Feinman, "Nutrition Education: A Questionnaire for Assessment and Teaching," *Nutrition Journal* 4, no. 1 (2005): 2.

2. F. B. Hu et al., "Dietary Fat Intake and the Risk of Coronary Heart Disease in Women," *New England Journal of Medicine* 337, no. 21 (1997): 1491–99.

3. M. Pollan, *In Defense of Food: An Eater's Manifesto* (New York: Penguin Press, 2008).

4. M. U. Jakobsen et al., "Major Types of Dietary Fat and Risk of Coronary Heart Disease: A Pooled Analysis of 11 Cohort Studies," *American Journal of Clinical Nutrition* 89, no. 5 (2009): 1425–32; P. W. Siri-Tarino et al., "Meta Analysis of Prospective Cohort Studies Evaluating the Association of Saturated Fat with Cardiovascular Disease," *American Journal of Clinical Nutrition* 91, no. 3 (2010): 535–46; P. W. Siri-Tarino et al., "Saturated Fat, Carbohydrate, and Cardiovascular Disease," *American Journal of Clinical Nutrition* 91, no. 3 (2010): 502–9.

5. American Diabetes Association, "Nutrition Recommendations and Interventions for Diabetes 2008," *Diabetes Care* 31, Supplement 1 (2008): S61-78.

6. A. Rabinovich, *The Yom Kippur War: The Epic Encounter That Transformed the Middle East* (New York: Schocken Books, 2004), 56.

7. American Diabetes Association, "Nutrition Recommendations and Interventions for Diabetes 2013," *Diabetes Care* 36, supplement 1 (2013): S12–32.

8. N. Teicholz, *The Big Fat Surprise: Why Butter, Meat & Cheese Belong in a Health Diet* (New York: Simon & Schuster, 2014).

9. G. M. Reaven, "Role of Insulin Resistance in Human Disease," *Diabetes* 37 (1988): 1595–607.

10. E. J. Fine, C. J. Segal-Isaacson, R. D. Feinman et al., "Targeting Insulin Inhibition as a Metabolic Therapy in Advanced Cancer: A Pilot Safety and Feasibility Dietary Trial in 10 Patients," *Nutrition* 23, no. 10 (2012): 1028–35.

11. W. B. Kannel and T. Gordon, "Diet and Regulation of Serum Cholesterol, Section 25," in *The Framingham Study: An Epidemiological Investigation of Cardiovascular Disease* (Washington, DC: National Heart, Lung, and Blood Institute, 1970).

Chapter 1: Handling the Crisis

1. F. Hahn, M. R. Eades, and M. D. Eades, *The Slow Burn Fitness Revolution: The Slow Motion Exercise That Will Change Your Body in 30 Minutes a Week* (New York: Broadway Books, 2003).
2. E. C. Westman, S. D. Phinney, and J. Volek, *The New Atkins for a New You: The Ultimate Diet for Shedding Weight and Feeling Great Forever* (New York: Simon & Schuster, 2010).
3. M. R. Eades and M. D. Eades, *Protein Power* (New York: Bantam Books, 1996).
4. J. S. Volek and S. D. Phinney, *The Art and Science of Low-Carbohydrate Living* (Charleston, SC: Beyond Obesity, 2011).
5. R. D. Feinman, M. C. Vernon, and E. C. Westman, "Low Carbohydrate Diets in Family Practice: What Can We Learn from an Internet-Based Support Group," *Nutrition Journal* 5 (2006): 26.
6. S. Somers, *Eat Great, Lose Weight* (New York: Crown, 1997).
7. R. C. Atkins, *Dr. Atkins' New Diet Revolution* (New York: Avon Books, 2002).
8. R. C. Atkins, *New Diet Revolution.*

Chapter 2: Whaddaya Know?

1. American Diabetes Association, "Nutrition Recommendations and Interventions for Diabetes 2008."
2. American Diabetes Association, "Nutrition Recommendations and Interventions for Diabetes 2013."
3. American Diabetes Association, "Standards of Medical Care in Diabetes—2012," *Diabetes Care* 35, supplement 1 (2012): S11–63.
4. American Diabetes Association, "Standards of Medical Care in Diabetes—2010," *Diabetes Care* 33, supplement 1 (2010): S11–61.
5. A. Keys, "Diet and Blood Cholesterol in Population Survey: Lessons from Analysis of the Data from a Major Survey in Israel," *American Journal of Clinical Nutrition* 48, no. 5 (1988): 1161–65.
6. U. Raynskov, *The Cholesterol Myths: Exposing the Fallacy That Cholesterol and Saturated Fat Cause Heart Disease* (Washington, DC: NewTrends Publishing, 2000); G. Taubes, *Good Calories, Bad Calories* (New York: Alfred A. Knopf, 2007); A. Colpo, *The Great Cholesterol Con* (Morrisville, NC: Lulu Press, 2006).
7. A. Keys, "Coronary Heart Disease in Seven Countries," *Annals of Internal Medicine* 73, no. 2 (1970): 356.
8. N. Teicholz, *The Big Fat Surprise*; U. Raynskov, *The Cholesterol Myths*; G. Taubes, *Good Calories, Bad Calories*; G. Taubes, "The Soft Science of Dietary Fat," *Science* 291 (2001): 2536–45; U. Ravnskov et al., "LDL-C Does Not Cause Cardiovascular Disease: A Comprehensive Review of the Current Literature," *Expert Review of Clinical Pharmacology* 11, no. 10: 959–970.
9. K. Sarri and A. Kafatos, "The Seven Countries Study in Crete: Olive Oil, Mediterranean Diet or Fasting?," *Public Health Nutrition* 8, no. 6 (2005): 666.
10. N. Teicholz, *The Big Fat Surprise.*
11. C. E. Forsythe et al., "Limited Effect of Dietary Saturated Fat on Plasma Saturated Fat in the Context of a Low Carbohydrate Diet," *Lipids* 45, no. 10 (2010): 947–62; C. E.

Forsythe et al., "Comparison of Low Fat and Low Carbohydrate Diets on Circulating Fatty Acid Composition and Markers of Inflammation," *Lipids* 43, no. 1 (2008): 65–77; J. S. Volek et al., "Dietary Carbohydrate Restriction Induces a Unique Metabolic State Positively Affecting Atherogenic Dyslipidemia, Fatty Acid Partitioning, and Metabolic Syndrome," *Progress in Lipid Research* 47, no. 5 (2008): 307–18.

12. T. McLaughlin et al., "Is There a Simple Way to Identify Insulin-Resistant Individuals at Increased Risk of Cardiovascular Disease?," *American Journal of Cardiology* 96, no. 3 (2005): 399–404.

13. F. B. Hu et al., "Dietary Fat Intake and Risk of Coronary Heart Disease in Women."

Chapter 3: The First Low-Carbohydrate Revolution

1. G. Willis, *Lincoln at Gettysburg: The Words That Remade America* (New York: Simon & Schuster, 1992).

2. J. A. Brillat-Savarin, *The Physiology of Taste: Or Meditations on Transcendental Gastronomy*, trans. M. F. K. Fisher (New York: Harcourt Brace Jovanovich, 1978).

3. R. C. Atkins, *New Diet Revolution*.

4. G. Taubes, "What If It's All Been a Big Fat Lie?," *New York Times Magazine*, July 7, 2002.

5. G. Taubes, *Good Calories, Bad Calories*.

6. *Fat Head*, directed by Tom Naughton (Burbank, CA: Morningstar Entertainment, 2009), DVD.

7. M. Pollan, *In Defense of Food*.

8. N. Teicholz, *The Big Fat Surprise*.

9. G. D. Foster et al., "A Randomized Trial of a Low-Carbohydrate Diet for Obesity," *New England Journal of Medicine* 348, no. 21 (2003): 2082–90.

10. G. D. Foster et al., "Low-Carbohydrate Diet for Obesity."

11. P. Leren, "The Oslo Diet-Heart Study. Eleven-Year Report," *Circulation* 42, no. 5 (1970): 935–42; P. Leren et al., "The Oslo Study: CHD Risk Factors, Socioeconomic Influences, and Intervention," *American Heart Journal* 105, no. 5 part 2 (1983): 1200–6.

12. O. Paul et al., "A Longitudinal Study of Coronary Heart Disease," *Circulation* 28 (1963): 20–31.

13. B. V. Howard et al., "Low-Fat Dietary Pattern and Weight Change Over 7 Years: The Women's Health Initiative Dietary Modification Trial," *Journal of the American Medical Association* 295, no. 1 (2006): 39–49; B. V. Howard et al., "Low-Fat Dietary Pattern and Risk of Cardiovascular Disease: The Women's Health Initiative Randomized Controlled Dietary Modification Trial," *Journal of the American Medical Association* 295, no. 6 (2006): 655–66; L. F. Tinker et al., "Low-Fat Dietary Pattern and Risk of Treated Diabetes Mellitus in Postmenopausal Women: The Women's Health Initiative Randomized Controlled Dietary Modification Trial," *Archives of Internal Medicine* 168, no. 14 (2008): 1500–11.

Chapter 4: Basic Nutrition: Macronutrients

1. M. Eades, "The Bad Fat Brothers," The Blog of Michael R. Eades, M.D., https://protein power.com/drmike/2007/04/23/the-bad-fat-brothers.

2. J. LeFanu, *The Rise and Fall of Modern Medicine* (New York: Carroll & Graf, 1999).

3. G. Taubes, *Good Calories, Bad Calories*.

4. N. Teicholz, *The Big Fat Surprise*.
5. M. U. Jakobsen et al., "Major Types of Dietary Fat and Risk of Coronary Heart Disease: A Pooled Analysis of 11 Cohort Studies," *American Journal of Clinical Nutrition* 89, no. 5 (2009): 1425–32; P. W. Siri-Tarino et al., "Meta-analysis of Prospective Cohort Studies Evaluating the Association of Saturated Fat with Cardiovascular Disease," *American Journal of Clinical Nutrition* 91, no. 3 (2010): 535–46; P. W. Siri-Tarino et al., "Saturated Fat, Carbohydrate, and Cardiovascular Disease," *American Journal of Clinical Nutrition* 91, no. 3 (2010): 502–9.
6. B. J. Brehm, "A Randomized Trial Comparing a Very Low Carbohydrate Diet and a Calorie-Restricted Low Fat Diet on Body Weight and Cardiovascular Risk Factors in Healthy Women," *Journal of Clinical Endocrinology and Metabolism* 88, no. 4 (2003): 1617–23.
7. S. Borghjid and R. D. Feinman, "Response of C57B1/6 Mice to a Carbohydrate-free Diet," *Nutrition and Metabolism* 9, no. 1 (2012): 69; B. Ahrén and A. J. Scheurink, "Marked Hyperleptinemia After High-Fat Diet Associated with Severe Glucose Intolerance in Mice," *European Journal of Endocrinology* 139, no. 4 (1998): 461–67; M. S. Winzell and B. Ahrén, "The High-Fat Died-Fed Mouse: A Model for Studying Mechanisms and Treatment of Impaired Glucose Tolderance and Type 2 Diabetes," *Diabetes* 53, suppl. 3 (2004): S215–19.
8. S. Klein and R. R. Wolf, "Carbohydrate Restriction Regulates the Adaptive Response to Fasting," *American Journal of Physiology* 262, no. 5 (1992): E631–36.
9. H. A. Harper, *Review of Physiological Chemistry*, 8th ed. (Los Altos, CA: Lange Medical Publications, 1961).
10. D. W. Martin et al., *Harper's Review of Biochemistry*, 20th ed. (Los Altos, CA: Lange Medical Publications, 1985).

Chapter 5: An Introduction to Metabolism

1. J. M. D. Olmsted, *Claude Bernard and the Experimental Method in Medicine* (New York: Abelard-Schuman, 1952): 76.
2. F. G. Young, "Claude Bernard and the Discovery of Glycogen: A Century of Retrospect," *British Medical Journal* 5033, no. 1 (1957): 1431–37.
3. G. F. Cahill, Jr., "Starvation in Man," *New England Journal of Medicine* 282, no. 12 (1970): 668–75.

Chapter 6: Sugar, Fructose, and Fructophobia

1. K. L. Stanhope et al., "Consuming Fructose-Sweetened, Not Glucose-Sweetened, Beverages Increases Visceral Adiposity and Lipids and Decreases Insulin Sensitivity in Overweight/Obese Humans," *Journal of Clinical Investigation* 119, no. 5 (2009): 1322–34.
2. M. A. Lanaspa et al., "Endogenous Fructose Production and Metabolism in the Liver Contributes to the Development of Metabolic Syndrome," *Nature Communications* 4 (2013): 2434.
3. R. D. Feinman and E. J. Fine, "Fructose in Perspective," *Nutrition and Metabolism* 10, no. 1 (2013): 45.
4. G. Taubes and C. K. Couzens, "Big Sugar's Sweet Little Lies," *Mother Jones*, 2012.

Chapter 7: Saturated Fat: On Your Plate or in Your Blood?

1. C. E. Forsythe et al., "Limited Effect of Dietary Saturated Fat on Plasma Saturated Fat in the Context of a Low-Carbohydrate Diet," *Lipids* 45, no. 10 (2010): 947–62.

2. C. E. Forsythe et al., "Comparison of Low Fat and Low Carbohydrate Diets on Circulating Fatty Acid Composition and Markers of Inflammation," *Lipids* 41, no. 1 (2008): 65–77; J. S. Volek et al., "Dietary Carbohydrate Restriction Induces a Unique Metabolic State Positively Affecting Artherogenic Dyslipidemia, Fatty Acid Partitioning, and Metabolic Syndrome," *Progress in Lipid Research* 47, no. 5 (2008): 307–18; J. S. Volek et al., "Carbohydrate Restriction Has a More Favorable Impact on the Metabolic Syndrome Than a Low Fat Diet," *Lipids* 44, no. 4 (2009): 297–309.

3. C. E. Forsythe et al., "Limited Effect of Dietary Saturated Fat."

4. S. K. Raatz et al., "Total Fat Intake Modifies Plasma Fatty Acid Composition in Humans," *Journal of Nutrition* 131, no. 2 (2001): 231–34.

Chapter 8: Hunger: What It Is, What to Do About It

1. B. F. Skinner, *About Behaviorism* (New York: Knopf, distributed by Random House, 1974).

2. R. D. Feinman and E. J. Fine, "Non-equilibrium Thermodynamics and Energy Efficiency in Weight Loss Diets," *Theoretical Biology and Medical Modelling* 4 (2007): 27.

Chapter 9: Beyond "A Calorie Is a Calorie": An Introduction to Thermodynamics

1. S. W. Angrist and L. G. Hepler, Order and Chaos: Laws of Energy and Entropy (New York: Basic Books, 1967), 215.

2. J. Hirsch et al., "Diet Composition and Energy Balance in Humans," *American Journal of Clinical Nutrition* 67, no. 3 (1998): 551S–55S.

Chapter 10: Diabetes

1. E. C. Westman and M. C. Vernon, "Has Carbohydrate-Restriction Been Forgotten as a Treatment for Diabetes Mellitus? A Perspective on the ACCORD Study Design," *Nutrition and Metabolism* 5 (2008): 10.

2. E. C. Westman, W. S. Yancy, Jr., and M. Humphreys, "Dietary Treatment of Diabetes Mellitus in the Pre-insulin Era (1914–1922)," *Perspectives in Biology and Medicine* 49, no. 1 (2006): 77–83.

3. D. J. Jenkins et al., "Effect of a Low-Glycemic Index or a High-Cereal Fiber Diet on Type 2 Diabetes: A Randomized Trial," *Journal of the American Medication Association* 300, no. 23 (2008): 2742–53.

4. E. C. Westman et al., "The Effect of a Low-Carbohydrate, Ketogenic Diet Versus a Low-Glycemic Index Diet on Glycemic Control in Type 2 Diabetes Mellitus," *Nutrition and Metabolism* 5 (2008): 36.

5. W. S. Yancy et al., "A Low-Carbohydrate, Ketogenic Diet to Treat Type 2 Diabetes," *Nutrition and Metabolism* 2 (2005): 34.

6. I. M. Stratton et al., "UKPDS 50: Risk Factors for Incidence and Progression of Retinopathy in Type II Diabetes over 6 Years from Diagnosis," *Diabetologia* 44, no. 2 (2001): 156–63.

Chapter 11: Metabolic Syndrome: The Big Pitch

1. G. M. Reaven, "Role of Insulin Resistance in Human Disease," *Diabetes* 37 (1988): 1595–607; G. Reaven, "Syndrome X: 10 Years After," *Drugs* 58, no. 1 (1999): 19–20.
2. G. M. Reaven," Role of Insulin Resistance"; G. M. Reaven, "The Metabolic Syndrome: Requiescat in Pace," *Clinical Chemistry* 51, no. 6 (2005): 931–38.
3. J. S. Volek and R. D. Feinman, "Carbohydrate Restriction Improves the Features of Metabolic Syndrome. Metabolic Syndrome May Be Defined by the Response to Carbohydrate Restriction," *Nutrition and Metabolism* 2 (2005): 31.

Chapter 12: The Medical Literature: A Guide to Flawed Studies

1. M. C. Gannon and F. Q. Nuttall, "Control of Blood Glucose in Type 2 Diabetes without Weight Loss by Modification of Diet Composition," *Nutrition and Metabolism* 3 (2006): 16.
2. R. D. Feinman and E. J. Fines, "Perspective on Fructose."
3. G. A. Bray et al., "Effects of Dietary Protein Contention, Weight Gain, Energy Expenditure, and Body Composition During Overeating: A Randomized Controlled Trial," *Journal of the American Medical Association* 307, no. 1 (2012): 47–55.
4. G. R. Norman and D. L. Steiner, *PDQ Statistics*, 3rd ed. (Hamilton, Ontario: B. C. Decker, 2003).
5. D. Colquhoun, *Lectures on Biostatistics* (London: Oxford University Press, 1971), http://www.dcscience.net/Lectures_on_biostatistics-ocr4.pdf.
6. H. Wainer, *Medical Illuminations* (Oxford: Oxford University Press, 2014).
7. L. J. Appel et al., "Effects of Protein, Monounsaturated Fat, and Carbohydrate Intake on Blood Pressure and Serum Lipids: Results of the OmniHeart Randomized Trial," *Journal of the American Medical Association* 294, no. 19 (2005): 2455–64.

Chapter 13: Observational Studies, Association, Causality

1. S. Weinberg, *Dreams of a Final Theory*, 1st ed. (New York: Pantheon Books, 1992).
2. S. Mukherjee, *The Emperor of All Maladies: A Biography of Cancer* (Waterville, ME: Thorndike Press, 2010).
3. J. LeFanu, *The Rise and Fall of Modern Medicine* (New York: Carroll & Graf, 1999).
4. J. LeFanu, *The Rise and Fall of Modern Medicine.*
5. L. E. Cahill et al., "Prospective Study of Breakfast Eating and Incident Coronary Heart Disease in a Cohort of Male US Health Professionals," *Circulations* 128, no. 4 (2013): 337–43.
6. S. Mukherjee, *The Emperor of All Maladies*, 246.

Chapter 14: Red Meat and the New Puritans

1. M. Pollan, *In Defense of Food.*
2. R. Stein, "Daily Red Meat Raises Chances of Dying Early," *Washington Post*, March 24, 2009.
3. R. Sinha et al., "Meat Intake and Mortality: A Prospective Study of Over Half a Million People," *Archives of Internal Medicine* 169, no. 6 (2009): 562–71.
4. D. K. Layman et al., "A Reduced Ratio of Dietary Carbohydrate to Protein Improves Body Composition and Blood Lipid Profiles during Weight Loss in Adult Women," *Journal of Nutrition* 133, no. 2 (2003): 411–17; D. K. Layman et al., "Dietary Protein and Exercise Have Additive Effects on Body Composition during Weight Loss in

Adult Women," *Journal of Nutrition* 135, no. 8 (2005): 1903–10; M. P. Thorpe et al., "A Diet High in Protein, Dairy, and Calcium Attenuates Bone Loss over Twelve Months of Weight Loss and Maintenance Relative to a Conventional High-Carbohydrate Diet in Adults," *Journal of Nutrition* 138, no, 6 (2008): 1096–100; P. J. Douglas et al., "Protein, Weight Management, and Satiety," *The American Journal of Clinical Nutrition* 87, no. 5 (2008): 1558S–61S; P. J. Douglas et al., "Role of Dietary Protein in the Sarcopenia of Aging," *The American Journal of Clinical Nutrition* 87, no. 5 (2008): 11562S–66S.

5. R. Sinha et al., "Meat Intake and Mortality."

6. A. Pan et al., "Red Meat Consumption and Risk of Type 2 Diabetes: 3 Cohorts of US Adults and an Updated Meta-analysis," *The American Journal of Clinical Nutrition* 94, no. 4 (2011): 1088–96.

7. A. Pan et al., "Changes in Red Meat Consumption and Subsequent Risk of Type 2 Diabetes Mellitus: Three Cohorts of US Men and Women," *Journal of the American Medical Association Internal Medicine* (2013): 1–8.

8. R. D. Feinman, "Red Meat and Type 2 Diabetes Mellitus," *Journal of the American Medical Association Internal Medicine* 174, no. 4 (2014): 646.

Chapter 15: The Seventh Egg: When Studies Defy Common Sense

1. S. Ebrahm et al., "Shaving, Coronary Heart Disease, and Stroke: The Caerphilly Study," *American Epidemiology* 157, no. 3 (2003): 234–38.

2. L. Djoussé et al., "Egg Consumption and Risk of Type 2 Diabetes in Men and Women," *Diabetes Care* 32, no. 2 (2009): 295–300.

Chapter 16: Intention-to-Treat: What It Is and Why You Should Care

1. D. Newell, "Intention-to-Treat Analysis: Implications for Quantitative and Qualitative Research," *International Journal of Epidemiology* 21, no. 5 (1992): 837–41.

2. S. Hollis and F. Campbell, "What Is Meant by Intention to Treat Analysis? Survey of Published Randomized Controlled Trials," *BMJ* 319, no. 7211 (1999): 670–74.

3. G. D. Foster et al., "Weight and Metabolic Outcomes after 2 Years on a Low-Carbohydrate versus Low-Fat Diet: A Randomized Trial," *Annals of Internal Medicine* 153, no. 3 (2010): 147–57.

4. "Comparison of Current NSLP Elementary Meals vs. Proposed Elementary Meals," Hunger-Free Kids Act of 2010, The White House, 2010, https://obamawhitehouse .archives.gov/sites/default/files/cnr_chart.pdf.

Chapter 17: The Fiend That Lies Like Truth

1. H. Wainer, *Medical Illuminations* (Oxford: Oxford University Press, 2014).

2. M. C. Gannon and F. Q. Nuttall, "Control of Blood Glucose in Type 2 Diabetes."

3. V. Hainer et al., "A Twin Study of Weight Loss and Metabolic Efficiency," *International Journal of Obesity and Related Metabolic Disorders* 25, no. 4 (2001): 533–37.

4. G. C. Smith and J. P. Pell, "Parachute Use to Prevent Death and Major Trauma Related to Gravitational Challenge: Systematic Review of Randomized Controlled Trails," *BMJ* 327, no. 7429 (2003): 1459–61.

Chapter 18: Nutrition in Crisis

1. U. Ravnskov, *The Cholesterol Myth: Exposing the Fallacy That Cholesterol and Saturated Fat Cause Heart Disease* (Washington, DC: New Trends Publishing, 2000); U. Ravnskov, "Cholesterol: Friend or Foe?"
2. R. D. Feinman and J. S. Volek, "Carbohydrate Restriction as the Default Treatment for Type 2 Diabetes and Metabolic Syndrome," *Scandinavian Cardiovascular Journal* 42, no. 4 (2008): 256–63.
3. A. Dahlqvists, *LCHF-blogg* (blog), 2014.
4. H. Monery, "Dr. Gary Fettke's 'Officially Cautioned,'" *The Examiner*, November 13, 2016.
5. W. Willett, personal communication to the author.

Chapter 19: Cancer: A New Frontier for Low-Carbohydrate

1. E. J. Fine, R. D. Feinman et al., "Targeting Insulin Inhibition as a Metabolic Therapy in Advanced Cancer: A Pilot Safety and Feasibility Dietary Trial in 10 Patients," *Nutrition* 28, no. 10 (2012): 1028–35.

Chapter 20: The Future of Nutrition

1. J. P. Ioannidis, "Meta-Research: The Art of Getting It Wrong," *Research Synthesis Methods* 1 (2010): 169–84; J. P. Ioannidis, A. Tatsioni, and F. B. Karassa, "Who Is Afraid of Reviewers' Comments? Or, Why Anything Can Be Published and Anything Can Be Cited," *European Journal of Clinical Investigation* 40, no. 4 (2010): 285–87; R. Horton, "Offline: What Is Medicine's 5 Stigma?," *The Lancet* 385 (2015): 1380; M. Angell, *Science on Trial* (New York: W. W. Norton & Co., 1996); R. Feinman and S. Keough, "Ethics in Medical Research and the Low-Fat Diet-Heart Hypothesis," *Ethics in Biology, Engineering and Medicine* 5, no. 2 (2014): 149–59.
2. E. J. Fine, C. J. Segal-Isaacson, R. D. Feinman et al., "Targeting Insulin Inhibition as a Metabolic Therapy in Advanced Cancer: A Pilot Safety and Feasibility Dietary Trial in 10 Patients," *Nutrition* 23, no. 10 (2012): 1028–35.

INDEX

Note: Page numbers followed by "f" refer to figures. Page numbers followed by "t" refer to tables.

ABOUT THE AUTHOR

RICHARD DAVID FEINMAN is a professor of cell biology at the State University of New York Downstate Medical Center in Brooklyn, New York, where he has been a pioneer in incorporating nutrition into the biochemistry curriculum. A graduate of the University of Rochester and the University of Oregon (PhD), Dr. Feinman has published numerous scientific and popular papers. Dr. Feinman is the founder and former coeditor-in-chief (2004–2009) of the journal *Nutrition and Metabolism*. His current research interest is in the application of ketogenic diets to cancer.

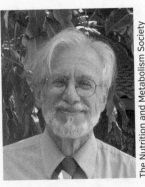

The Nutrition and Metabolism Society

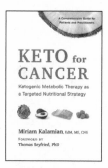
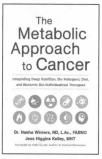
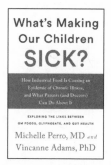
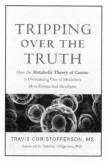
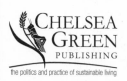

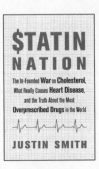
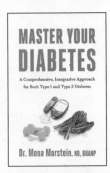
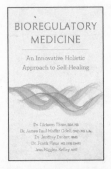
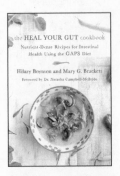
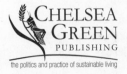